PSYCHIATRY
in American Life

PSYCHIATRY
in American Life

edited by Charles Rolo

Essay Index Reprint Series

BOOKS FOR LIBRARIES PRESS
FREEPORT, NEW YORK

The editor wishes to thank the following for permission to reprint copyrighted material:

The Atlantic Monthly for articles by Clemens E. Benda, Stanley Cobb, Robert Coles, Mignon McLaughlin, O. Hobart Mowrer, Peter B. Neubauer, Mortimer Ostow, Philip Rieff, John R. Seeley, Greer Williams.

Atlantic–Little, Brown for "The Language of Pundits" from CONTEMPORARIES by Alfred Kazin, © 1961 by Alfred Kazin.

Esquire for "Psychotherapy in America — The Contemporary Scene" by Brock Brower. First published in *Esquire* Magazine, July, 1961, under the title "Who's In Among the Analysts," © 1961 by *Esquire, Inc.*

Harper & Row, Publishers, for "Freud and Jung," originally published as two chapters entitled "Science and Emotion" and "Jung and Comedy," from THE HIDDEN REMNANT by Gerald Sykes, Copyright by Gerald Sykes 1962.

INTERNATIONAL STANDARD BOOK NUMBER:
0-8369-2424-X

LIBRARY OF CONGRESS CATALOG CARD NUMBER:
76-156711

PRINTED IN THE UNITED STATES OF AMERICA
BY
NEW WORLD BOOK MANUFACTURING CO., INC.
HALLANDALE, FLORIDA 33009

Acknowledgment

THIS VOLUME grew out of a Special Supplement of the *Atlantic Monthly*, *Psychiatry in American Life*, which I edited in collaboration with my former colleagues on the *Atlantic*. I wish to record my thanks to all of them, in particular to Edward Weeks, who brought to the project his enthusiasm, editorial acumen, and several valuable contributors; and to Emily Flint, who shared with me the hazards involved in editing the manuscripts of savants.

C. R.

Contents

PSYCHIATRY
in American Life

The Freudian Revolution

CHARLES ROLO

———•———

THE most revolutionary changes are changes in man's basic beliefs about himself. Three such revolutions have occurred in Western thought in the past five hundred years — the Copernican, the Darwinian, and the Freudian — and they have successively dealt shattering blows to man's pride. Copernicus dethroned man from the center of the universe. Darwin challenged his sense of divinity by tracing his descent to the animal kingdom. And Sigmund Freud, the first cartographer of the unconscious, punctured his conviction that the conscious mind was master of man's fate. "I belonged," Freud justly said, quoting the poet Hebbel, "to those who have profoundly troubled the sleep of mankind."

Freud's discoveries are the original source of most of the developments and issues discussed in this symposium. For, as W. H. Auden wrote after Freud's death in 1939, "To us he is no more a person/Now but a whole climate of opinion." Freud first used the word psychoanalysis in print in 1896, and the first major statement of his doctrine, *The Interpretation of Dreams*, appeared on November 4, 1899. Thus psychoanalysis is roughly the same age as the twentieth century. What were its origins and what does it represent in terms of the cultural history of Western society?

Psychoanalysis derives from and draws together two sharply antithetical traditions. In many respects, it is a child of nineteenth-century science and hence descended from the rationalism of the Enlightenment. On the other hand, some of its crucial insights into human nature and its emphasis on man's inner life reflect the vision of the Romantic poets and philosophers of the nineteenth century. In this respect, it belongs to the broad cultural movement which rejected and undermined the dominant ideas of the Enlightenment and the utopianism of Victorian science — the view that man was essentially "good" and perfectible, that reason was the sovereign power, and that increasing mastery over nature spelled "inevitable progress."

The influences which worked directly on Freud were in the main scientific. As a medical student in Ernst Brücke's institute at the University of Vienna, Freud absorbed a "physicalist psychology" strongly colored by Darwinism and the theories of Hermann Helmholtz. This physiology viewed the human body as a system of atoms moved by forces acting in accordance with Helmholtz's principle of the conservation of energy — the principle that the sum of forces remains constant in every isolated system. It held that science, through lack of knowledge, was forced to distinguish between various kinds of forces — mechanical, electrical, magnetic, and so on — but that progress would eventually show that there were only two: attraction and repulsion.

In the field of psychology, Freud acknowledged the influence of G. T. Fechner, a disciple of T. F. Herbart, whose theories were expounded in a textbook in use in Freud's last year at secondary school. Herbart developed a dynamic psychology of unconscious processes some seventy years before Freud; indeed, so many of his ideas foreshadow Freudian concepts that one wonders whether he was not a genius born too soon to find the world ready for his message. Herbart's central thesis was that it must eventually be possible to describe mental processes in terms of scientific laws, and he dreamed of a "mathematical psychology." Fechner worked in this direction by trying to incorporate into psychology, as Freud was to do later, Helmholtz's principle of the conservation of energy. Thus, to sum up these influences, nineteenth-century science contributed the framework into which Freud tried to fit his psychological discoveries. This framework was deterministic and materialistic, strongly oriented towards physics and evolutionary biology.

In contrast, the *content* of psychoanalysis relates it to the Romantic movement, which was gathering momentum when Freud was born in 1856. The superior power of passion over reason, the fateful duality of man's nature, exploration of "the night side" of life — these were central concerns of the Romantic poets and philosophers. Wordsworth, for example, was preoccupied with the hidden sources of his thoughts and "unknown modes of being." Coleridge referred to "the unconscious" and to "the twilight realms of consciousness." Eduard von Hartmann's *Philosophy of the Unconscious*, published in Berlin in 1869, achieved considerable celebrity. C. G. Carus, whose book *Psyche: The Development of the Soul* made a strong impression on Dostoevski, asserted an intimate relationship between conscious and unconscious life. Freud himself observed that Schopenhauer's concept of "unconscious will" was roughly equivalent to the instincts in the mind

— the "id" — as seen by psychoanalysis. Schopenhauer also hinted at the relationship developed by Freud between repression and mental illness: "In the resistance of the [unconscious] will against allowing what is distasteful to come into the illumination of the intellect lies the place where insanity can break into the mind." "Schopenhauer," said Thomas Mann, "as psychologist of the will is the father of all modern psychology. From him the line runs, by way of the psychological radicalism of Nietzsche, straight to Freud and the men who built up his psychology of the unconscious and applied it to the mental sciences."

In Freud, the two traditions I have sketched were forged into what amounts to a synthesis. Working in the spirit of the Enlightenment and modern science, Freud found the encouraging conception of human nature handed down by the Enlightenment sadly inadequate by reason of its failure to recognize the tremendous and inescapable power of irrational, unconscious forces in the life of mankind. But Freud's therapeutic credo — summed up in the famous formula "Where id was, there ego shall be" — is the statement of a rationalist who believes that knowledge is power; who affirms that man, by bringing repressed ideas into consciousness, can make them amenable to the control of reason and stop or at least mitigate their ravages. Indeed, Jung's principal objection to Freudianism is that it is far too rationalistic and insensitive to the creative possibilities of the irrational.

Certainly Freud's emphasis on the relative weakness of the conscious mind and on the terrifying power of biological drives does not lead to any cult of irrationalism; it is designed, rather, to furnish reason with a more realistic strategy in its eternal conflict with the instincts. And though he is generally considered a pessimist, Freud sounds a note of hope about the outcome of this conflict. In *The Future of an Illusion,* there is this moving passage: "The voice of the intellect is a soft one, but it does not rest until it has gained a hearing. Ultimately, after endlessly repeated rebuffs, it succeeds. This is one of the few points on which one may be optimistic about the future of mankind, but in itself it signifies not a little. And one can make of it the starting point for yet other hopes. The primacy of the intellect certainly lies in the far, far, but still probably not infinite, distance." In sum, the Freudian revolution represents an agonizing reappraisal of the rationalist tradition and an attempt to revise it drastically — but in order to salvage rather than destroy it.

Up to this point, I have been discussing psychoanalysis in terms of cultural history. I have not forgotten that, as the late Gregory Zilboorg put it, "psychoanalysis was born out of medical necessity." Dr. Zilboorg, an eminent psychoanalyst, was referring to the fact that when Freud was a young neurologist, medicine still had no real understanding of mental disorders and no effective treatment for them. In *A History of Medical Psychology,* Dr. Zilboorg and his collaborator, Dr. George W. Henry, wrote: "After a century of effort — inaugurated by Pinel — spent in studying the forms of mental illness, after fifty years of persistent attempts to exact from the anatomy of the central nervous system and from general physiology an answer to the question of what mental disease was, medical psychology could not help but sense and admit that it did not know the answer." However, as Freud put it, "psychoanalysis did not gush forth from the rock nor fall from heaven." Among the outside influences which put Freud on the track that led to psychoanalysis were Jean Charcot's celebrated demonstrations of hypnotism in Paris; the experiments of Ambroise-Auguste Liébault and Hippolyte Bernheim, who, at a clinic in Nancy, were treating hysterics by using hypnotism combined with suggestion; and the report of Freud's friend and mentor Dr. Josef Breuer that a patient of his showed marked improvement after being put in hypnosis and urged to talk about what was oppressing her — a method the patient christened the "talking cure."

The irony in this drama of momentous discovery is that Freud, who ended the impasse in the treatment of mental illness and revolutionized psychiatry, had become a doctor only "through being compelled to deviate from my original purpose." This purpose was to be a scientist who could devote himself without distractions to understanding and perhaps solving some of the great riddles of nature. Indeed Freud, though until the very end of his life he spent most of his day analyzing patients, was not primarily interested in the therapeutic aspects of psychoanalysis. His "consuming passion," his "tyrant" was psychology; and in his later years, he ventured audaciously into "metapsychology" and became a system-builder seeking to impose order on the chaos of reality. "The triumph of my life," he wrote, "lies in my having, after a long and roundabout journey, found my way back to my earliest path."

It is not surprising, then, that Freud should have expressed great concern lest psychoanalysis be "swallowed up by medicine." He felt strongly that psychoanalysts should not necessarily be doctors of medicine. He believed that psychoanalysis needed within its ranks men whose primary bent was for psychology and men with a sensitivity to the arts, and he feared that insistence on a medical degree might turn some of them away. For Freud the importance of psychoanalysis lay not in its therapeutic benefits but rather in its contributions to knowledge.

Thus psychoanalysis has several aspects which need to be distinguished. On its practical side, it is a specialized diagnostic and therapeutic technique within the domain of psychiatry, the branch of medicine that concerns itself with mental disturbances. It is also an organized body of theories about human behavior, and as such is a part of psychology. How much of it meets the scientific canons of formal psychology is a matter of dispute. Its influence on clinical psychology has been large, but the gulf between psychoanalysis and so-called academic psychology remains wide, even though members of each discipline have studied the other.

Thirdly, psychoanalysis has distinct philosophic implications, which were developed in Freud's later work and have been elaborated by his interpreters. Freud chose to deny that psychoanalysis was committed to any particular *Weltanschauung*, but it has in effect become a doctrine with its own philosophy. All of these aspects of psychoanalysis — along with popular misconceptions, and with heresies and innovations, some of which may represent progress — have contributed to the cultural revolution which one is forced to call Freudian, even though there is much in it for which Freud was not responsible, much that would horrify him.

The impact of this revolution has been incalculably great in the United States. To an extent not paralleled elsewhere, psychoanalysis and psychiatry in general have influenced medicine, the arts and criticism, popular entertainment, advertising, the rearing of children, sociology, anthropology, legal thought and practice, humor, manners and mores, even organized religion. In fact, the long arm of the Freudian Revolution has reached into the Congress of the United States. Alarmed by the information that some nine million Americans suffer from serious mental troubles, the Congress, in 1955, passed an act authorizing an elaborate study of the nation's mental health. This unprecedented inquiry has resulted in the publication of eleven volumes, of which the most arresting is *Americans View Their Mental Health,* a survey which implicitly holds up to us a new character ideal — psychological man. As Philip Rieff has observed, three character ideals have successively dominated Western civilization: the political man of classical antiquity; then religious man; and from the Enlightenment to the present, economic man. Now it seems to be the turn of psychological man, who lives by insight, counting his satisfactions and dissatisfactions, studying his worries, watching over his mental health.

Several of the contributors observe that psychoanalysis, by force of circumstances, has in effect become a secular religion. This approach places many of the distressing aspects of the Freudian revolution in their proper perspective. The awful movies depicting quasi-miraculous psychoanalytic cures; the slick novels and dramas in which bad Daddy and possessive Mummy are the source of all evil; the cocktail party sages who have translated gossip into solemn psychoanalytic jargon — these and many other unattractive phenomena of our psychology-conscious age have their counterparts in the vulgarizations and corruptions to which religion has been subjected.

It would seem, indeed, that psychoanalysis is to some extent the victim of its own success. A good many of the complaints voiced against it betray excessive demands or expectations. People point to acquaintances not benefited by analysis as proof that its claims are not substantiated, but no responsible analyst has asserted that worthwhile results are achieved in more than 50 to 60 per cent of the cases. One hears, too, gibes about the conduct and competence of analysts which seem to be based on the assumption that the profession should be immune to human fallibility; it is inevitable that there should be a certain number of defective analysts, just as there are mediocre surgeons, bad doctors, and errant priests.

Of course, there is much in the theory, practice, and cultural repercussions of modern psychiatry that invites debate or criticism. My hope is that this symposium will help to illuminate certain segments of this large and controversial subject. In this connection, it might be helpful to say something about the principles which have guided the editing.

In the first place, I have deliberately sought diversity of opinion. Various schools of thought are represented, and the reader must be prepared for divergent and even sharply conflicting points of view. I have even included an essay — that by Professor O. Hobart Mowrer, an eminent psychologist — which asserts that psychoanalysis has been a total failure as a therapy, and in the sphere of human conduct has fostered a destructive irresponsibility. I myself find this thesis refuted by overwhelming evidence, but Professor Mowrer has stated succinctly and forcibly what may loosely be termed "the case against psychoanalysis," and I feel his essay merits a place in the symposium.

One of the liabilities of an editorial approach which seeks diversity of opinion is that exposure to disagreement may leave certain readers uncomfortably perplexed. But it is healthier, surely, to be left perplexed than to be "brainwashed," and there must be many who will consider it an asset that this volume, taken as a whole, has no doctrinal axe to grind. It does not seek to preach any kind of orthodoxy or win converts for any particular psychiatric gospel. It seems to me innocent, too, of a charge which is frequently leveled at practitioners of modern psychiatry, psychoanalysts in particular — the charge that they tend to suffer from complacency and arrogance. In the pages which follow, there is a vigorous and varied body of criticism and self-criticism. In fact, it is the critical spirit which prevails.

The editor of a symposium dealing with any specialized or technical subject and aimed at the intelligent layman has to pursue an elusive goal: a combination of authority and readability. If, taken as a whole, this volume comes somewhere near to achieving that combination, it should serve a useful purpose. It does not presume to address itself to the specialist, who has a hard time anyhow keeping up with the formidable output of professional journals; nor, on the other hand, does it dispense any of the popular brand of "inspirational psychiatry."

The contributors are a varied and interesting lot. Six are doctors of medicine engaged in the practice and/or teaching of psychiatry or psychoanalysis. One is something of a rarity — a Freudian psychoanalyst without a medical degree. One is a professor of psychology. The remaining eight are informed laymen with varying degrees of involvement in psychiatry — for their credentials, see Notes on the Contributors (page 244).

In conclusion, it might be appropriate to mention briefly the editor's personal convictions about modern psychiatry. They can be summed up as follows: It is surely beyond doubt today that modern psychiatry is able to help people who could not previously be helped; anyone who has seen the transformation it can bring about in a painfully disordered child is apt to be impatient with the chronic scoffers. It has emphasized the role of love in normal development and has produced a new awareness of the importance of childhood, a greater generosity of spirit toward the needs of the child. It has provided man with ways and means of deepening his understanding of himself and of his basic problems as a culture-building animal. In sum, it represents, perhaps, a crucial breakthrough in man's pursuit of self-knowledge and self-realization.

PART I

Theory and Practice

Mind and Body — The Development of Psychosomatic Medicine

STANLEY COBB, M.D.

———•———

THE ills imposed on man's body by the conspiracies of fate have for ages been a subject for poets and storytellers. The Greeks drew tragic nets about their heroes; situations forced them to commit acts for which they suffered mentally and physically. To the Greeks, gods, demons, and witches were responsible. Two thousand years later, Shakespeare saw the play of human passions more subtly. He described their effects on the bodies of his characters and even suggested psychotherapy in some instances.

In more modern times, physicians describe emotional reactions in their professional writings: "Under the active stage of anger, the following train of phenomena will be displayed in greater or lesser strength. The heart now aroused beats quickly and forcibly and the blood, rushing impetuously to the head and surface, the brain becomes heated, the face flushed, the lips swollen, the eyes red and fiery, the skin hot, and literally may it be said we burn with anger."

This quotation is from a wonderful book by Dr. William Sweetser, professor of the Theory and Practice of Physik at Bowdoin Medical School. It was published in 1843, and the title runs: *Mental Hygiene, or an Examination of the Intellect and Passions, designed to illustrate their Influence on Health and Duration of Life.* Speaking of the effect on the digestive tract, Dr. Sweetser goes on to say: "Anger destroys the appetite, and checks or disorders the function of digestion. Let one receive a provocation in the midst of his dinner, and the food at once loses all its relish for his palate. Dr. Beaumont, who had under his charge a man with a fistulous opening into his stomach, so that the interior of this organ could actually be inspected, remarked that anger, or other serious mental emotions, would sometimes cause its inner, or mucous coat, to become morbidly red, dry and irritable; occasioning, at the same time, a temporary fit of indigestion."

William Beaumont was the real pioneer in the physiology of the emotions. He was an army surgeon stationed at Fort Crawford on the upper Mississippi River during the 1820s. One day a Canadian trapper who had been shot through the stomach was brought to him. He grasped this opportunity with great imagination, and there in the wilderness made his classic observations of the physiology of digestion. A hundred and twenty years later, in New York, Dr. Harold Wolff found a similar patient. With modern techniques he elaborated the findings of his backwoods predecessor and wrote his own classic, *A Man and His Stomach.* Sweetser's collection of observations and stories concerning the effects of the passions was the forerunner by almost a century of Helen Flanders Dunbar's scholarly and closely documented *Emotions and Bodily Changes,* published by the Macy Foundation in New York in 1935. During that century, medicine took on the form of a science. Between 1850 and 1900, however, the great light shed on medicine by advances in bacteriology, microscopical pathology, and surgery cast its shadow on psychology. The majority of physicians were convinced that all diseases would be explained by the microscope; little was heard of psychology and the possibility that thoughts and feelings might affect medical symptoms.

Syphilis as a cause of mental disease had been suspected for a century. The discovery of its true role in psychiatry was both a great advance in knowledge and an inhibitor of psychological understanding. "Softening of the brain" (also known as paresis, general paralysis of the insane, and dementia paralytica) was one of the first clinical pictures to be recognized. Until the recent development of antibiotic treatment, this disease caused much of the severe mental illness that sent patients to fill our mental hospitals. There were many theories as to the cause of paresis. Early in the nineteenth century, "the strain of modern life" was blamed, as well as head injury, excessive mental work, alcohol, and venery. Syphilis was not seriously considered as a cause until 1857. Clinical observation and inoculation experiments made it seem probable. The Wassermann test for syphilis, developed in 1906, clinched the matter by showing that over 90 per cent of patients with paresis had "positive" reactions. If any doubters remained after this, they had to accept the discovery at the Rockfeller Institute by Hideyo Noguchi and Joseph W. Moore in 1913 of the syphilitic spirochete within the brain. This was a research triumph and made investigators hopeful that all mental disorders could eventually be explained by bacterial and other injuries to the brain. Such speculation consolidated a group of psychiatrists and neurologists into a mechanistic school, and they were later to be known as "organicists." They had little interest in psychology.

In the years around 1900, psychiatry was stirring in its cocoon. For a hundred years it had been a special branch of medicine, the first "specialty," because of the necessity of isolating lunatics in asylums. This was a matter of taking queer and disturbing persons out of an unsympathetic population; it had little to do with treatment. A few dedicated physicians gave their lives to caring for these unfortunates, but too many of the retreats were little better than prisons. Emil Kraepelin in Berlin made the first effective move to bring order out of chaos. By keen clinical observation he grouped the inmates of the madhouse into different categories of disease and was thus able at least to prognosticate with some accuracy whether or not a patient might recover. But his interests were largely in clinical classification and the changes found in the brains of those who died in asylums. He was greatly impressed by the findings in paresis. He did not think that life experience, personality, and emotions had much to do with mental breakdown. In short, he did not believe in psychogenesis. Finally, his authoritative systematization was opposed by some younger psychiatrists, who dubbed it "Imperial German Psychiatry."

The group that gradually formed in opposition to the organicists was composed of good thinkers who understood the problems of the psychiatric hospitals but had broad training outside. Psychiatry had been bound within the walls of the asylums. Sigmund Freud, Eugen Bleuler, and Pierre Janet in Europe, and James Jackson Putnam, Adolf Meyer, and Morton Prince in America gave impetus to the stirrings for liberation. Their dynamic psychological interpretations of mental illness began the great change which took a large part of the practice of psychiatry out of the mental hospitals and into private offices and general hospitals.

As early as 1908 Meyer wrote, "And it has become my conviction that the development of some mental diseases are rather the results of peculiar mental tangles than the results of any coarsely appreciable and demonstrable brain lesions or poisonings." His comprehensive view of psychiatry was developed largely between 1900 and 1915. It was probably influenced by Freud's ideas concerning the neuroses, but Meyer worked in large hospitals in New York and Baltimore and was more concerned with severe mental illness. His concept of the psychological precipitants preceding mental breakdown permeated all modern psychiatric thought. No psychiatrist would now study a patient without trying to learn about his pre-psychotic personality. Meyer preached the necessity for gathering all pertinent facts about a patient and seeing not only the mental disorder in the patient but the "he" or the "she" who is ill, in the setting of his or her life situation. The importance of psychogenesis was emphasized not as *the* cause of mental disorder but as one factor to be carefully weighed. Facts concerning heredity, body build, medical status, and any other relevant data were all considered.

Freud's contributions between 1893 and 1938 have gone beyond medicine and have affected the thinking of most literate people. His approach was clinical, bringing in the techniques of free association and prolonged day-by-day analysis. His important concepts included the theory of drives, repression, the unconscious mechanisms, the development of sexuality in infant and adult, and ego development. Indeed, a rich and disturbing set of ideas! The simplest of them, the idea of unconscious motivation, was profoundly distasteful to the Victorian culture of the century's end, with its worship of individualism, will power, and Protestant morals.

> It matters not how strait the gate,
> How charged with punishments the scroll,
> I am the master of my fate:
> I am the captain of my soul.
> — W. E. HENLEY (1849-1903)

In fact, one of the charges against Freud and all dynamic psychiatrists has been that by explaining abnormal human behavior they condone it and take away from a person his choice and "free will." It is charged that they take away responsibility and preach fatalism. This is a strange accusation against those who are trying to free men from their unconscious motivations and compulsions; against earnest physicians who are striving to help their patients toward maturity and toward altruistic behavior in place of their childish, neurotic, and antisocial reactions.

The dynamic psychology of today can be traced back to several lines of thought, dimmed between 1847 and 1900 but emerging slowly as the end of the century approached. Those who used hypnotism and studied the effects of suggestion and emotions on the bodily functions did something to keep psychological theory alive. Oliver Wendell Holmes, between 1856 and 1885, wrote three novels which showed much insight into personal problems, forecasting some of Freud's contributions. *Elsie Venner* is the best known but least psychological. *A Mortal Antipathy* and *The Guardian Angel* describe quite specifically the effects of frights in infancy upon the later development of personality. Holmes explained that he considered his colleagues in the medical profession not yet ready to accept such psychological truths; therefore, he did not publish them in medical journals but disguised them in what he called his "medicated novels." In 1899 James Jackson Putnam lectured to the Massachusetts Medical Society on "Not the Disease Only, But Also the Man." But in 1911 he was booed at a meeting of the American Neurological Association for supporting Freud's views. Few medical scientists were brave enough to challenge the ascendancy of the microbe.

Charles Darwin in 1873 had written a remarkable book describing emotional reactions as important biological phenomena, but it was not until forty years later that two great physiologists contributed to this field. Ivan Pavlov, in Russia, studying memory and learning in dogs, added much to our knowledge of emotions. Walter B. Cannon, in Boston, was the first investigator who seriously took up the problem of the physiology of the emotions. He made it a profound and respected study and published in 1915 a book entitled *Bodily Changes in Pain, Hunger, Fear and Rage: An Account of Recent Researches into the Function of Emotional Excitement.*

Nowadays, when every educated person absorbs some of the concepts of psychogenesis and motivation in general reading, and when every medical student learns something more about them in his early psychiatric studies, it does not seem possible that Kraepelin so recently dominated psychiatry. The fact that psychological reactions could be dynamic was made brutally clear to hundreds of army medical officers during World War I. They saw with their own eyes that violent emotion could and did cause severe illness. Soldiers were brought to hospitals with paralyzed limbs, deafness, blindness, and loss of the sense of smell — all caused psychologically and curable by psychotherapy. Even such medical diseases as goiter and diabetes were seen to be precipitated by fear and stress. These medical officers returned to become practicing doctors, but they had learned about psychogenesis and were willing to listen sympathetically to the teachings of psychiatry and physiological psychology.

Gradually a body of knowledge was brought together that became known as psychosomatic medicine. This is not a specialty, but rather a comprehensive approach to medical problems which attempts to evaluate all pertinent factors, particularly the personal and psychological. It is a field for research where medicine and psychiatry meet. The term "psychosomatic" was first used by Johann Christian Heinroth in 1818. In the late 1920s it was reborn, and reached maturity when the American Psychosomatic Society was formed in 1944. What it is all about is best explained by giving a case history:

Mary Brown, age twenty-five, came to the Massachusetts General Hospital because of painful finger tips on both hands and small ulcerations of the skin. She was suffering from Raynaud's disease, a disorder of the nervous system and blood vessels in which the small arteries of the hands and feet undergo periods of abnormal contraction. This shuts off the blood supply to the fingers and toes: they turn white, and later, as the arteries relax, they become swollen, blue, and painful. If the periods of arterial spasm are prolonged, the lack of oxygen supply through the blood may cause death of the tissues. The first result is ulceration of the skin, which may spread dangerously. The attacks are usually brought on by cold or anxiety. The best treatment is to avoid cold and anxiety, but this is often impossible, so surgery is employed. The nerves that cause contraction of the responsible arteries are cut near their exit from the spinal canal. With these nerves gone, spasm of the arteries becomes impossible.

Mary looked worn and older than her years but still retained a certain youthful attractiveness of manner. She was from a fishing village in Rhode Island, where her Portuguese parents had brought her up in a decaying Yankee culture. She had always been a somewhat reserved child and had kept her sorrows to herself. Her mother died when she was twelve, and she immediately took over responsibility for her three younger brothers. Two years later her father remarried, and this she seemed to accept as inevitable. At the age of seventeen she married a man several years her senior; in spite of squabbles, they had a good relationship and much happiness. At the end of a year a son was born, and for the next two years things went along reasonably well. Then she learned that her husband had been already married, that the former wife was alive, and that her marriage was illegal. The shock was great, but she decided to stick by her husband. They planned to separate for a year, during which he would get a divorce from his wife and then legally marry our patient. During the year of separation he visited her too frequently and impregnated her. The plans for divorce and remarriage failed. He went to California; she tried to produce an abortion by taking ergot, but failed. She then married a local fisherman, much older than herself, because she needed a home and protection. Shortly after this marriage, the second son was born and rather gracefully accepted by the new husband. Three years later she became pregnant by her second husband.

Her first attack of Raynaud's disease occurred under the following circumstances: She had been for some time carrying on a correspondence with her first huband. Her second husband had forbidden the continuance of this correspondence, but she kept it up despite him. On a hot summer day in 1933 she had gone to the post office expecting to find a letter from her first husband. When she asked for the mail, the clerk said that her husband had already called and taken it. This meant to her that her second husband had found the letter; she believed that he would have recognized it and opened and read it, and she feared the consequences. She knew that he would resent the tone in which her first husband wrote to her. Badly frightened and trembling, she went out into the street. There she formed a plan of drowning herself and the two boys. At the same time, while she was trembling, fearful, and forming ideas of suicide, she noticed that the little finger of her right hand was numb and white, while the fingernail was blue. She was so struck by this change in her little finger that she went into a grocery store and showed it to an acquaintance. This condition continued for about an hour.

Her second attack occurred on the ensuing day: her husband revealed to her that he did, indeed, have the intercepted letter. She demanded that he give it to her; he refused; there was a scene. Then she went to the dock with her two sons, intending to drown herself and them. As she stood by the water with her two boys, she noticed that the fingers of both her hands had become blue and painful. Then a man appeared on the dock, preventing her from carrying out the suicidal plan. She again attempted abortion by taking medicine, but failed and went through with the pregnancy.

After this sudden onset, the patient had such attacks almost daily. During the first year of her disease, only the finger tips were affected, but later the disturbance extended to the mid-palm of both hands and simultaneously involved both feet, which became white and cold but did not ache as did her hands. During these attacks, the patient felt her heart pounding hard and fast, and there was a dull pain in that region. Her fingers became puffy, her feet swelled, and she had increasing difficulty in closing her fists. Small ulcerations appeared on the finger tips. The attacks occurred when she was cold, tired, hungry, or scared.

Three years after the onset of her disease, operations were performed, first on the vasomotor nerves of the left hand, and then on the right. The ulcerations healed as the circulation improved, and the attacks of arterial spasm ceased. She was referred to one of the hospital psychiatrists for psychotherapy.

No one knows why some persons are susceptible to Raynaud's disease and others are not. Heredity may play a part. Cold is the usual stimulus that sets off an attack, but in cases like that of Mary Brown the precipitating cause is clearly psychological. A thought leads to fear, and the emotion sets off nerve impulses which traverse the nerve to the artery and make it shut down. A normal and necessary function has gone too far. In this case, the surgeon stopped the ulceration and pain in the fingers. The psychiatrist and social worker carried on to relieve the emotional stress.

From the practical standpoint, psychosomatic medicine is the field where the psychiatrist can work with the medical man or surgeon for the benefit of the patient. By its very nature, it is a cooperative and comprehensive endeavor and would lose all meaning if it became a specialty. Physicians and investigators have become increasingly interested in the field because in the last twenty years new facts have been found in neurology, psychology, and physiology that increase our understanding of complicated human situations.

I remember clearly the meeting at which the American Psychosomatic Society was organized. Dr. Meyer was present and much interested, although he could not approve of the name "psychosomatic." He said rightly that the two words "psyche" and "soma," even joined in one, emphasize our illogical way of thinking of mind and body as different and separate things. Twenty years later we are still working to educate physicians to look on a man as a unified organism. Thinking of mind and body as separate leads to slighting one or emphasizing the other, to the detriment of the patient.

Take, for example, a man who has been seen by me over the last ten years — a carpenter and cabinetmaker of seventy-five, retired, living alone, and with decreasing ability to continue his beloved handicraft. He complained of "restless legs" at night, with muscular spasms and jerks that interfered with sleep. There was a history of old injury to the neck, and x-ray revealed a severe destructive arthritis of the cervical vertebrae. This explained the symptoms, but not their great exaggeration whenever his loneliness and fear of the future made him tense and anxious. He was helped by a combined treatment of orthopedic neck traction, careful use of drugs, and occasional psychiatric talks. But he kept coming back to me in frantic doubt, asking, "Doctor, is this physical, or am I neurotic?" My painstaking explanation always improved the situation for a while. I told him that he certainly had arthritis of the neck and explained how anxiety made muscular tension and therefore increased his spasms and insomnia. Nevertheless, he kept shopping around for new opinions. These usually took one side or the other and lacked a comprehensive grasp of his illness. So they confirmed his neurotic fear, and he kept coming back to me with the same old question.

If we, as practicing physicians, do not really believe in the unity of mind and body, we either think, "There's nothing wrong with this patient; it's only nerves," or we ride the other hobby and in our enthusiasm for psychotherapy overlook symptoms that could be relieved medically. It is common to find a patient incapacitated because a small pain he could well live with — if given understanding support — has been built up into much suffering. I never saw a patient with purely imaginary pain.

A large part of the art of medicine is understanding people. In 1927 Francis W. Peabody, in his lecture at the Harvard Medical School on "The Care of the Patient," declared that the art of medicine and the science of medicine were not antagonistic but supplementary. He pointed out that the physician who attempts to take care of a patient while neglecting his emotional life is as unscientific as the investigator who neglects to control all the conditions that may affect his experiment. Dr. Peabody died before psychosomatic medicine was talked about, but like all great and benevolent physicians, he understood it well.

In many medical communities, young physicians are taught to spend more time collecting data from the laboratory than quietly listening to the patient tell his story in his own words. There has been a tendency to leave this to the psychiatrist — an unfortunate result of specialization, because many patients who seem to have straightforward medical or surgical problems are not given a chance to talk. Psychiatrists have learned to listen. Leaders in the teaching of psychosomatic medicine, such as Franz Alexander, Carl Binger, and Felix Deutsch, have done much to keep the human side of medicine alive. But the emphasis has been to teach this art as part of psychiatry. It should be a cornerstone of medicine.

Psychotherapy in America
—The Contemporary Scene

BROCK BROWER

THAT first couch was of horsehair. Pyramided high with pillows. *Berggasse 19, Wien IX.* ("After the — well, later when the Professor is no longer with us," the porter said one day to the poet H.D. on her way to her fifty-five-minute "hour," "they will call it Freudgasse." They never did.) For some of his taller patients, it was almost too short, and their feet under the couch rug nearly touched the glowing porcelain stove set narrowly in the corner. From the other corner, behind the couch's hard, slightly elevated headpiece, came the cigar smoke and the fatherly voice. "Today we have tunneled very deep. You have discovered for yourself what I discovered for the race." Around him, the sublimations of a frustrated archaeologist: Greek amphorae, Assyrian and Egyptian statuettes, and other tiny, ancient totems, set all in a row. And over the couch — on the wall usually reserved nowadays for the stark probe of a favored pair of analytical eyes — a large steel engraving of the Temple of Arnak, for this was the only consulting room in the history of psychoanalysis where it was not possible to hang on that wall an honorific portrait of the analyst's chosen St. Analyst.

Now, fifty years after the official founding of the faith at the already quarrelsome Nuremberg Congress, there is a hagiology to choose from — the Professor himself or the Diaspora: Alfred Adler, C. G. Jung, Otto Rank, Wilhelm Stekel, Sandor Ferenczi, Frieda Fromm-Reichmann, Karen Horney, Erich Fromm, Wilhelm Reich, Harry Stack Sullivan, *inter alios* — and under these framed and glaring imagos, the weak, often shattered egos of the modern personality, couchant on foam rubber, squat, brass-booted legs, inclined pillows, dark leather, or the whole tweedy spectrum of upholsterers' fabrics. The couch is now long enough, low enough, wide enough and fashionable enough for everybody, and some heretical analysts will even let their patients sit right straight up in a chair. ("It's easier to lie down on a couch and discuss the past than to sit up in a chair and face the future!" claim the Adlerians in their incorrigible optimism.) The propagation of the faith has forced the quaint Viennese stove to give way to thermostatically controlled professional care in barren, green-walled office apartments from Beverly Hills to Central Park West, and where the Professor's old rug once lay — at the foot of the horsehair couch, neatly folded for each of his incoming patients — is now most often a plastic sheath to protect the fabric from muddy heels.

America is the most psychoanalyzed country in the world. And this despite Freud's own firm conviction that America was basically a mistake: "A gigantic mistake, it is true, but nonetheless a mistake." He never trusted the future of his ideas here. Even though America gave psychoanalysis its first public recognition when Freud delivered his famous lectures at Clark University in 1909, he constantly worried about the mixing of "the pure gold of psychoanalysis" with the dross of lesser psychotherapies in this much-too-democratic country. He once made a scathing prediction that the major use America would make of his theories would be to incorporate them into its advertising.

His distrust, however, is really a classic instance of an analysis that ended too soon. He saw the patient for less than a month during 1909, gave an absurd diagnosis ("America is already threatened by the black race. And it serves her right. A country without even wild strawberries!"), and departed, blaming his brief stay for everything from his intestinal trouble to the deterioration of his handwriting. But he left the analysand in a far worse state, for he never understood what a deep conflict his dark theories of unconscious instinctual drives — sex, aggression, and death — would set up in the American psyche with its root optimism and surface gleam. When the force of his discoveries began to be felt here, partially in the Twenties, profoundly in the late Forties, he became a cathected object in our system unconscious, charged with all the unsettled emotions directed toward the analyst by a patient forced too quickly to abandon cherished defenses. There has never yet been any release. We are more dependent than we know on the Stern European Father, who left us, then died before any real adjustment was found between his grim truths about the individual unconscious and our open, conscious, Constitutional pursuit of happiness. Nowadays, if he visited us, we'd be more careful. We'd probably see to it that he was flown out to a patch of wild strawberries in a comfortable helicopter, just to make *sure* he'd like us, stay over, take Our Case.

But too late, the psychic damage is done, and it has caused chaos in the American psychoanalytic situation ever since.

The pure gold of psychoanalysis, for instance, has to be kept under constant guard by an encoiled organizational dragon called the American Psychoanalytic Association. (There are so many non-Freudians who would steal it and make of it amulets of their own.) The association is the largest, most respected group of analysts in the country, with about one thousand full members on its rolls and a like number in training. It holds the dominant and more or less ordained position here, but its hegemony is constantly under challenge from rival schools and theories that seem to proliferate as fast as any single deviating analyst can lengthen his own shadow into an institution. To some extent, these splinter groups are simply reflections of older quarrels from Vienna — the Jungians, the Adlerians, the Rankians, *et al.* — but the splintering has gone much finer than that at times. There is now available, by appointment, psychobiologic therapy, Gestalt therapy, directive therapy, nondirective therapy, conditioned-reflex therapy, rational therapy, psychopuppetry, psychotherapy by reciprocal inhibition, and *family* therapy, to name only a few of the odder persuasions that still lie outside the orgone box.

Of course, these splinter groups are found only on the outer fringe of what one Freudian calls "the red-light district of psychoanalysis." At the heart of that district exist a number of other, lesser dragons that operate almost in institutional parallel with the American Psychoanalytic Association, offering journals, clinics, theories of character structure, training analyses, certifications, internal quarrels, and mutual referrals entirely their own. Their adherents often picture themselves as serving Freud — if not to the exact letter of *The Ego and the Id,* at least in the proper analytic spirit — *better* than the Freudians.

"I revere Freud," says Isidore Portnoy, M.D., a member of the neo-Freudian Karen Horney Clinic. "For his discovery of the unconscious. For his work with dreams, free association — the fact that nothing can be disconnected inside the human being. For his search for truth — nobody has carried on as sincere, tenacious and determined a search for truth as Freud did. But some of the Freudians — not *all* of them, but *some* of them — make too strict a business out of analysis. You're supposed to be neutral toward the patient, but it's impossible to be neutral. If the analyst isn't aware of that, his big toe's going to be aware of it and fall asleep on him. Then you're supposed to be a mirror for the patient. Well, some of the Freudians — not *all* of them, but *some* of them —just use that to hide behind. They're too neurotic themselves to face the patient, to get involved with another Self."

This kind of talk, of course, is anathema to the orthodox Freudians. One of them has referred to Karen Horney's theories as "psychoanalysis of the Sanka genre," presumably psychoanalysis with all the caffeine taken out, so it doesn't disturb the patient's rest on the couch. But it's quite typical of how Freud is often evoked by a non-Freudian, not as *the* god, at least as a central figure in the psychoanalytic pantheon. A lay analyst will justify his nonmedical status by quoting Freud's enthusiasm for lay analysis; a Reichian will go back to Freud's original libido theory as proof of the existence of orgones; or Norman O. Brown in *Life Against Death* will reinterpret Freud to prove that "The proper aim of psychoanalysis is the diagnosis of the universal neurosis of mankind, *in which psychoanalysis is itself a symptom and a stage."*

Perhaps the best that can be said of the reigning anarchy in psychotherapy is that, despite their differences, most analysts are honestly in search of a common good: the improvement of the analytic relationship. And, in the end, the private association between analyst and analysand is what really matters. "In psychoanalysis, you check your degree at the door," remarks Charles Winick, associated with the New York Postgraduate Center of Psychotherapy. "The only thing that counts is the application of a relationship." Joost A. M. Meerloo, M.D., keeps one rule foremost in approaching each new patient: "Distrust every label, but ask for the case history." All analysts believe that every case is intensely individual, that flexibility is needed in order to reach the patient, and that the analytic relationship is arduous, exacting, and full of pitfalls. "I can't think of any harder work than being an analyst," one of them explains. "At the end of the day, I'm utterly exhausted. The only thing that comes close to it is being *in* analysis."

It seems astonishing then that analysts would make the work all that much harder by quarreling so often among themselves, but though the major betrayals and ostracisms are decades old, factionalism continues. Some of the younger analysts believe it is on the decline: "We're more in communication with each other today." But as the first generation of American-born analysts, they have the advantage of a kind of Innocence Abroad in the overly Europeanized intellectual atmosphere of psychoanalysis. They don't bear the scars of old religious wars. Other critics see factions as actually having hardened, grown more formal. "The day they start publishing in each other's journals or crossing institutional boundaries in making patient referrals," says Dr. Winick, "then I'll say they're free of factionalism." One analyst gave a classic riposte when he was asked in a public discussion how on earth, with all the various schools, a poor layman was to know which one was the right school? He fixed the questioner with a nondirective stare and said, "You're *obsessed* with rightness!"

The public has perhaps been even more obsessed with analysis itself, and the vulgarization of psychoanalysis has done its own share of psychic harm. It is one of the problems today that everybody — like Freud, but unfortunately without his genius — is constantly analyzing himself, and then, for good measure, his fiancée, his mother, his favorite poet, and his chief opposition. Analysts often find that it is one of the blocks their patients bring to the couch. "This incessant ruminating on the self is something I try to get my patients to work through *during* their analysis," says Dr. Portnoy. "It's what Shelley called 'the dark idolatry of self.' " Basically ludicrous, like sticking pins happily in one's own waxen image, it nevertheless points to an even larger problem — "the considerable danger," according to Rollo May, "that psychoanalysis and psychotherapy in general will become part of the neurosis of our day rather than part of the cure."

Fortunately the vogue for psychoanalysis as a "thing" appears to be on the wane. It was at its height just after the war, when a great many veterans used their G.I. Bill funds to study psychology, apparently hoping to find in it an answer to the regimentation of a society that looked as if it too had been taken over by the Army while they were away. In the early Fifties, the first thick volume of Ernest Jones's laborious and scholarly biography of Freud even became a freak best-seller.

Sales plummeted to more sensible figures, however, on

the next two volumes, which actually meant that they enjoyed "a more appropriate readership," according to publisher Arthur Rosenthal of Basic Books, Inc., "among
people seriously interested in the study of psychoanalysis,
instead of a lot of cocktail-party sophisticates looking for
new chatter." During the past four years, there has been
a highly reasonable leveling off in the situation. The influx
of students has remained static, and analysis itself has
come to be considered a much more private matter than it
once was. One mentions one's analyst, just to show *sang-
froid* about the relationship, but one doesn't go on and *on*
about him. Analysts themselves are approached at social
gatherings as something other than queer ducks that will
make the most fascinating quacks. One does *not* say, "I
met this head-shrinker at a party the other night, and
brother, was *he* disturbed!" In general, the analysts,
though they've lost what one of them calls "our narcis-
sistic glory," are much relieved by the change. "When I go
to a party, I don't get bothered by people who think I'm going to open my pocket and out will fall The Answer!"

And despite the "thing" that all the wrong people have
had about analysis, the broader general awareness has re-
dounded in many ways to the patient's benefit. He comes
much sooner to seek help, with a much more sophisticated
attitude toward the therapy he faces. "It used to be that a
person had to be paralyzed in a good part of his life before
he came to us," says Jacob A. Arlow, M.D., past president
of the American Psychoanalytic Association. "Now, much,
much sooner." Perhaps too often they come knowing too
much — "They've read Freud. Or about him. You have to
ignore that. They're just intellectualizing, which will get
them nowhere" — or expecting too much — "You have to
watch out for people with omniscient expectation. Either

you don't take them as patients, or you try to find why psychologically they *have* these expectations." Miracles simply don't happen, even on the smallest order. "The other day a patient got annoyed at me because I called attention to his cold," reports one analyst, "and asked him why he didn't try some nose drops. 'You're supposed to cure me of this,' he says. I can't even do that. What I can do is much closer to something another patient of mine said when we ended it. 'All analysis has done for me' — then he stopped because he realized he'd made a slip, revealed something about his attitude — 'What analysis has done for me is to help me begin to struggle.' That's it, right there. It can help a person begin to struggle." Many people, still far short of a breakdown but suffering acutely after some personal catastrophe, such as a divorce or a career failure, come for just this sort of help.

They do not come — as some critics of analysis carpingly imply — in childish search of a surrogate Dutch uncle. They are deeply disturbed, but disturbed in such a way that Freud would hardly recognize them as neurotics. They have none of the classic psychoneurotic symptoms, nor any of the violence, that distinguished Freud's famous cases, e.g., Dora, whose perverted sexual desires, directed toward her father, her father's mistress, and her father's mistress's husband, produced clearly hysterical symptoms; or the Wolfman, who during their first interview offered to bugger Freud and then defecate on his head. Analysts seldom encounter these extremes of behavior today; in fact, violent patients are becoming fewer and fewer even in the psychiatric wards. The present problem is overriding passivity. "A masochistic form of compliance," Dr. Meerloo describes it. "The ego is so weak, it can't defend itself." Outwardly, the neurotic's life pattern may appear to be reasonably normal, but inwardly he is made incredibly anxious, sometimes immobile, by a feeling of total dissatisfaction with his own life.

The complaints of these sufferers might be the street cries of the twentieth century. *I'm blocked. I'm drifting. I'm stuck, and I can't get out. I'm living with a stranger.* "They don't know the word, but what they mean is *alienation,*" says Dr. Portnoy. Their tribulation, however, goes much deeper than the intellectual's existential despair. Emotionally, the neurotic personality is at a loss to achieve its own identity. Sexual ambivalence is often part of the nightmare confusion in which the neurotic lives. It is responsible for the increasing number of homosexual patients analysts are encountering — "the ultra masochism, the ultra passivity," Dr. Meerloo describes the disorder — but it can also underlie a great many supposedly nonsexual life choices. "A patient comes to me with a career problem. Supposedly. He can't decide whether to go into chemistry or physics," says Dr. Arlow. "Then I begin to find that all his symbols, his feelings, about chemistry are feminine, and all his enthusiasms for physics are masculine. His real problem is his sexual role."

And although these patients are quiescent, almost too rational, they are much harder to reach and help than Freud's more violent patients. Dora broke off her analysis after only eleven weeks, but Freud already had come somewhat to grips with her hysteria. Now analysis may last as long as six to eight years — much to the distress of the analysts, by the way, who would honestly prefer a constant influx of new patients rather than the same old faces all the time.

Perhaps the most important fact to be noted from this glimpse of mental disorders is that the entire diagnostic character of the neurosis has altered since the late-nineteenth-century investigations into hysteria by Freud and Breuer. Neurosis is more passive, more complicated, and, most important of all, more pervasive of the whole personality structure than it was once recognized to be. The rude awakening for most analysts came during the late Forties, and ever since their shop talk has been mostly a series of subtler and subtler refinements on neurotic character structure. "We used to have a simple obsessional neurosis." (A Freudian speaking here, obviously.) "A person had to carry out a certain act, or else he felt anxious, and he could tell *himself* that something specific was disturbing him. But now we have obsessional *character*. A person's whole life has that quality of overly rigid compensation that once marked the single obsessional act, and he can't tell *what* is disturbing him." Against these fine points there have been some loud outbursts, from Erich Fromm and other "social neo-Freudians," protesting that neurosis is *of our time* rather than *of the individual personality;* but in general, those analysts who really keep shop continue the painstaking work of unraveling the individual tangle of human personality, and it seems more or less true that upon increasingly smaller and more delicate strands depends the measure of their success.

And to a great extent, this tight, long-haul, almost surgical approach is the measure of the analysts themselves. "There is no Freud, no Adler, no Jung in this country now," remarks Charles Winick. "The texture of these men differs entirely from that of the great men of the past. They may be better analysts. Frequently they are — much better analysts, in fact. But there are no giants in the field." There are some men who are mentioned always, and by everyone, regardless of allegiance, with respect —

among them, Franz Alexander, M.D., whose work in psychosomatic medicine brought about a small revolution in the healing arts, or Lawrence Kubie, M.D., who championed the teaching of psychoanalysis in the country's medical schools; or Erik H. Erikson, whose famous study of the child greatly extended general knowledge of ego psychology. But most of the leading analysts have earned their reputations in the name of the Great Names. For them, the truth has already been incarnate upon this earth. Their work has therefore been apostolic rather than messianic, and any catalogue of their achievements really amounts to a study of the extension of creeds.

And among the various sects, the Freudians still come first — by a long chalk. Not only are they more in number than all the other analysts put together, but they have also done the most thorough exegetical work on the doctrines of their teacher. They have concentrated on the ego, rather than on the id or superego, and the development of ego psychology, through a careful study of the ego defenses, has been their main emendation of classical Freudianism since Freud's death. Though a primer on the subject is impossible here, three general observations can be made that will perhaps bring its outlines into view:

(1) The ego, according to a definition offered by Anna Freud, can perhaps best be compared in its psychic function to the civil service in a modern state. "She pointed out," writes Charles Brenner, M.D., "that in a complex society the citizen must delegate many tasks to civil servants if he wants them done efficiently and to his own best interests. The creation of a civil service is therefore to the individual citizen's advantage and brings him many benefits which he is happy to enjoy, but at the same time he discovers that there are certain disadvantages also. The civil service is often too slow in satisfying a particular need of the individual and seems to have its own ideas of what is best for him, ideas that do not always coincide with what he wants at the moment. In a similar way the ego may impose delay on the id drives, may argue the claims of the environment against them, and even appropriate for its own use some of the energy of the drives by means of neutralization."

(2) If this, however, represents more or less the normal function of the ego, it is also true that, like any civil service, the ego can suffer from a number of bureaucratic ills. It may become so weak that it does nothing but shift papers around and sign its name in triplicate to documents that have no meaning at all. Or it may meet every crisis situation in a completely inadequate manner, following an old and erroneous routine, so ingrained that it can't be abandoned even in the face of the obvious catastrophes it causes. Or it may elaborate complicated office procedures that are actually designed to bury any real trouble or distress in the files or route them quickly to another bureau. These are the so-called ego defenses, which include such psychic mechanisms as *denial* ("Thus the subject matter of a repressed image or thought can make its way into consciousness on condition that it is *denied*" — Freud), *isolation* (a person will face complete knowledge of some personal disaster without feeling any emotional involvement whatsoever), or *projection* (a racial bigot will accuse the hated minority of all the darknesses he fears in himself).

(3) The problem of therapy then becomes *structural*. Neurosis cannot be treated by simply coring it out of the psyche, as if it were the lone bad spot in a basically sound apple. The classical Freudian belief that a neurotic could

be cured by making him aware of his unconscious desires and motivations — through the translation of dream symbols, free association, parapraxes, etc. — is a lost hope. A much more complex awareness is needed, an awareness on the analysand's part of all the evasions and defenses he has been employing to avoid facing his troubles. Therapy amounts to a restructuring of the ego — and, in many cases, since it has been pathetically weakened, a fortifying of the ego through the patient's identification with a stronger personality, i.e., the analyst — so that eventually the ego can deal efficiently and effectively as mediator between the id drives and the demands of the environment. In effect, the ego becomes a reformed and modernized civil service.

In the painstaking work on a body of theory for ego psychology, three names stand out, and very much together — Heinz Hartmann, M.D., the late Ernst Kris, and Rudolph M. Loewenstein, M.D. "They are the three dictators of ego psychology," says another Freudian. Among the three, Dr. Loewenstein's reputation as a dedicated analyst is particularly high, though Hartmann's is the name most often and most widely mentioned in Freudian circles. Ernst Kris, however, was the *rara avis*. A brilliant researcher and a vastly cultured Old European gentleman, he did not have a medical degree, and was one of the few "special members" of the American Psychoanalytic Association.

Studies in ego psychology often have a bizarre quality about them, as if they were jobs of precision tooling done on the worst of human crudities. Research offering further proof that the model of the defense of projection is the physical experience of defecation, carried over from childhood, might be taken as a typical piece of work.

It might also be taken as the perfect mark for the kind of attack that non-Freudians delight in leveling against ego psychology. Modeling projection on anality, according to non-Freudian polemics, is just what a Freudian *would* do. The idea offends in every way: it's too pat; it depends entirely on infantile sexuality, Freud's polymorphous perversity of the child, which simply isn't true; it's a mechanical explanation that's too abstract to be of any use in analysis; it's utterly defeatist, *dooming* a grown man to a childish pattern of behavior; and besides, on its face, it's perfect nonsense, isn't it? What the Freudians have been struggling to discover with their ego psychology, concludes any one of these bombasts, is what *we've* known for years, exactly what Our Leader discovered when he broke with Freud. Each of the schools believes it has grasped one simple truth that the Freudians miss in their blindness, and one index to these schools is what each of them believes that simple truth — immanent in ego psychology, of course, but hopelessly obscured — happens to be.

To the Adlerians, for instance, ego psychology is just a clever front for their holistic approach. "The holistic approach is now accepted by *everybody*," says Mrs. Danica Deutsch, executive director of the Alfred Adler Consultation Center and Mental Hygiene Clinic, casting an evil eye across Central Park at the East Side Freudians. "They all realize that a person is goal-directed. They all talk about a person's *life style*. A pity they forget where the phrase came from." It came from Alfred Adler, as indeed did a good many other concepts — screen memories, the inferiority complex, etc. — that have crept into psychoanalytic usage.

But present Adlerian techniques are about as analytically orthodox as a block party. The Adlerians are bent on rousing the neurotic to develop social interest. "An individual can only fulfill himself if he works within the society," says Mrs. Deutsch, "and his social interest is the yardstick of his mental health." Emphasis is placed particularly on the family, and therapy can strike the whole family at once, like the measles. If Tommy is recommended for treatment by his schoolteacher, he goes into Play and Art Therapy along with his brothers and sisters; his mother goes into Group Counseling for mothers; and his father should put in an appearance at evening Group Counseling for parents. The Adlerians have arrived at group therapy as "the natural result of man as a social being." They even have a Therapeutic Social Club, now in its fifth year (dancing, ping-pong, outings), where patients can meet one another and sometimes get married. (The best cure for a neurosis is to fall in love, Freud once said.)

There seems to be a feeling among the Adlerians that they gave forth truth, and now nobody stops around to see them any more. The Alfred Adler Clinic was one of the first of its kind in the country. "Other clinics asked us for our constitution," says Mrs. Deutsch proudly. "But now our waiting list of patients is shrinking. It's the fault of all the new private clinics opening up. It's the pills."

However, the Adlerians, who are still about two hundred and fifty strong in this country, are much better off than the Jungians or the Rankians. A careful search of the Yellow Pages, in fact, fails to uncover a Rankian much above a social worker, and if any Rankian organization exists, it is somewhere underground, recovering from the birth trauma. The Jungians are at least active enough to keep their objection to ego psychology vocally current. To wit: "The whole pattern of relatedness sets the result in analysis. In Freudian psychology, an unseen authority makes *ex cathedra* statements when the patient is lying there, open, helpless. In Jungian psychology, we are interested in the patient's genuine reactions. The goal is a relationship."

That relationship is built to last, too, for the Jungians keep their spirits up through a kind of clubbiness, in which all successful analysands share. Jung intends his system as an instrument for the psychological development of *normal* people as well as disturbed patients. After a minimum number of hours of analysis — "sometimes a hundred, usually rather more" — a patient may be recommended by the analyst for membership in an Analytical Psychology Club (New York, London, Zurich). At club meetings, there are lectures, discussion groups, seminars in Jungian psychology, which admittedly require some study to keep up with their intellectual demands. In 1960, the New York Analytical Psychology Club held a seminar under M. Esther Harding, M.D., the *doyenne* of New York Jungians, on "The Reconstruction of the Injured Archetypal Image," which was all very fine — if, as one Jungian pointed out, "you had enough libido for it."

The quarrel the Jungians have with Freudian psychology is that it is too narrow, too reductive. Certainly, they admit, the weakened ego is an ever-present problem — "The hospitals are full of people who are possessed by archetypal images, only without adequate ego to relate to them," says Edward Edinger, M.D. — but to be healthy even the strong ego must relate to something larger than itself. Neurosis is "a state of cosmic anxiety," brought about because "symbol systems don't contain people any more, psychologically." To be healthy and growing, the ego must relate to superpersonal elements in life, so that the individual himself becomes "rooted in a consciousness that contains symbols much bigger than his own ego."

It is a highly spiritual approach, best suited, according to Jung, to patients over thirty-five. However, the younger Jungians have managed to drop the age limit back to a point where there are even Jungian child psychologists.

Dr. Edinger estimates Jungian psychology in this country is about where Freudian psychology was forty years ago. "It's growing slowly," he says. "But it doesn't seem to be congenial with the radically extroverted American mind. Certainly there's no bandwagon."

On the other hand, the neo-Freudian approach of Karen Horney does seem remarkably compatible with the optimistic American temperament, and members of the American Institute for Psychoanalysis, though only a hundred strong, appear to believe they have overtaken ego psychology in one simple stride. "Ego? What is it? Nothing more nor less than the Self. We're happy about that because we've been working with it for years." However, Horney's Self is hardly the same entity as the Freudian ego. It is a much freer, more easily reversible proposition.

Certainly among the *émigrés* who openly challenged orthodox analysis in this country, Horney knew the largest success, having before her death transformed her personal cult into a lasting psychoanalytic movement. Others less fortunate have struggled along with their votaries, meeting sometimes bitter, sometimes ludicrous fates. One wholly respected sanctuary for the unorthodox is the William Alanson White Institute of Psychoanalysis, Psychiatry, and Psychology in New York. Here, a Ph.D may sit down with an M.D. without scandal on either side, and their sympathies, though probably basically Freudian, will be very much with any sound suggestion for a new approach to the analytic relationship. In this tolerant spirit, the White Institute has housed analysts of such relatively diverse convictions as White, Fromm, Frieda Fromm-Reichman, Clara Thompson, and, notably, Harry Stack Sullivan, whose theories of interpersonal relationships are perhaps the chief teaching at the institute. Most recently, it was a fellow of the institute, Rollo May, who brought national attention to a European innovation in psychoanalysis — existential analysis — and started a critical dialogue that, almost of its own accord, is turning into one movement, if not several.

Perhaps it is better to view existential analysis not as a movement but as a highly structured and persistent question. It comes upon the scene just when psychoanalysis is under attack from a number of outside critics who are no longer incensed, as in the Twenties, by its challenge to traditional values, but rather by the sterility—as they see it—of the current Freudian ethic. And possibly at the core of existential analysis lie the very self-doubts that some analysts must feel as this new attack mounts. After all, there are people on all sides of them who would have the future write them off as practitioners of an art that failed to heal, or a science that turned to myth.

"We are right in the center of an antipsychoanalytic period," one analyst explains. "Analysis has always been unattractive — financially, personally, socially, in every way — but precisely because we *do* have it now, and it *is* working, more people are beginning to see how hard and difficult it is. As Ernest Jones said, there's always going to be resistance to analysis unless it's diluted to some kind of easy, pastoral treatment."

The attack on the analysts has indeed spared them nothing. Their fees, their cures, their scientific intelligence, and their own mental health have all been questioned. Other therapies have been pitted against them. Group therapy, which began in the veterans hospitals as a way to help more people, is now extolled as a better way to help everybody. (Its fees now often equal, or even surpass, those of the analyst.) Medicines, particularly lysergic acid (LSD), have been offered as a substitute for analysis. Quicker, more certain, more scientific. "You know, it's all said rather gloatingly," one analyst points out. " 'Ah, you guys, you'll be out of there as soon as we get the right chemical!' But you show me a pill that's going to help a guy get along better with his wife, and then I'll say you've got something."

In light of this attack, there are two definitions of an analyst (both of them given by analysts) that might be taken as indicative of both the best and the worst of the present situation. The first defines an analyst as a *proletarian de luxe;* that is, a wage slave, who works by the hour, but at a very high rate. This is precisely the problem. An analyst can treat only a limited number of patients, and each of them must stay with him a long, long time at fees that range between fifteen and forty dollars per hour. This is painful to the patient, and also painful to the analyst, who would prefer that analysis be much shorter, less exacting, and more easily afforded. But apparently it cannot be, because, according to the second definition, an analyst is he who "dives deeper, stays down longer, and comes up dirtier" than any other therapist. And this is precisely the benefit. Over the long haul, analysis will bring about a change in the disturbed patient — "not what he expected probably, but nevertheless a real change" — that no other approach to man's whole being has yet been able to achieve.

Some will stoutly deny even this last, but in the face of such hostility, the analysts can be forgiven for falling back on their most invincible habit. They analyze the hostility.

"The public today reminds me of a patient who has just gotten over the first thrill of finding himself in analysis," says Dr. Portnoy. "Disillusionment is beginning to set in a little. Well, if the patient's got anything to him, he's going to get over that. He's going to come back with a much more knowing, more humble attitude. The same with the public. They're not going to throw analysis out just because it's hard work. Ways of searching for the truth aren't a dime a dozen, you know."

The Psychoanalytic Treatment Process

RUDOLPH WITTENBERG

FREUD made it clear early in his writings that the ideal analytic patient is somebody whose functioning in daily life is not too drastically impaired. In practical terms this means that there has to be enough cooperation to go to the daily analytic session, enough of a healthy core to tolerate the uncovering of useless neurotic defenses, enough strength to give up the dubious satisfactions of neurotic behavior, enough patience to wait for the emergence of the solid core inside the personality.

All this becomes apparent early in the treatment, when the patient is told to say anything that comes to his mind. Without any special preparation, the patient is asked to keep the control gates down for fifty minutes several times a week — to avoid censorship, concern with content and direction, indeed, all purposeful control of his speech. In short, he is asked to do the very opposite of what he has learned — *not* to choose what makes immediate sense or to keep watch over what he is saying.

Learning to abide by this basic rule — which, as a matter of fact, is the only rule of psychoanalysis — is part of the treatment process. Slowly the patient discovers that in free association, too, there is selection, a different order of continuity from the one he is accustomed to — that of the complicated structure of the preconscious and unconscious parts of the mind. He realizes that the sequence of free associations makes a kind of sense after all, that random thoughts and feelings, "left-field" memories, and seemingly wild impulses in due course begin to reveal a new dimension of the inner world. A person accustomed to acting on impulse discovers that in the analytic process nothing is acted on. This is one of the important safeguards in analysis which permits the giving up of conscious control over verbal communication: everything should be expressed, but nothing is acted out.

Another difficulty in learning to say anything that comes to mind is the fact that the analyst often does not respond to the patient's utterances. All of us are used to a certain pattern of communication in our lives. When we speak to somebody, we usually get a response. Hence the analyst's long silences can be disconcerting and even exasperating. The analyst usually has to listen for a long time before he can speak. This is not simply because, as in all situations, one has to understand before one can help; it is determined by the analytic process itself. The analyst is not there to react the way people usually do when we speak to them, but to remain open with all his senses, conscious and unconscious, to the associations of the patient.

The more unobtrusive the analyst remains, the better for the patient's flow of associations. The analyst listens with free-floating attention, absorbing and trying to put together the many pieces of the puzzle. He has been trained to associate to his patient's associations and to use his clinical judgment about when to intervene or to interpret.

Among the things that come to the patient's mind as he associates freely are his dreams. In a way they are the freest associations. Dreams have their own language, which cannot be translated into understandable, every-day meaning without a special dictionary. The dictionary is the patient's free associations, not the analyst's specu-lation or ramblings. Without the free associations, one does not know what events were used for the dream tap-estry; one cannot connect present and past, or understand what emotions relative to the analysis are being ex-pressed.

As the patient free-associates, as he relates dreams, the reasons for needing to cling to his fantasies will become apparent and the analyst can help him to see them with new eyes, aiding him to re-evaluate his experiences and to separate past from present.

It is therefore helpful if the patient's picture of the an-alyst is vague, and it is quite true that this picture encour-ages regression. But regression is one condition of re-experiencing, and it is the hub of the psychoanalytic method of treatment. The neurosis will unfold in the ana-lytic relationship — instead of with the patient's family and business associates. The situation is structured to achieve this end.

One of the aspects of the analytic relationship which encourages the reliving of experiences is the use of the couch. So much has been said about it — and it has been the source of so many jokes — that perhaps we should explain more fully just what its function is.

Historically, the use of the couch for therapeutic pur-poses is older than analysis. Dr. Josef Breuer, one of Freud's colleagues and early supporters, used it between 1880 and 1882 for inducing hypnosis in a now famous case of hysteria. The hypnosis resulted in the reproduction of hysterical symptoms in the doctor's office, and their subsequent disappearance. The patient named this treatment the "talking cure," and Breuer called it "catharsis," a then new method of psychotherapy. While he was developing psychoanalysis, Freud continued to use the couch, at first to facilitate hypnosis, which he originally thought of as an essential step, later to facilitate recollection, and still later because it was conducive to free association. He has also told us in his writings that he could think about what his patients were saying, and understand them better, if they did not search his face for answers to their troubles.

Thus the use of the couch is designed to facilitate the process of re-experiencing. It enables the patient to say anything that comes to his mind with less embarrassment than he would feel if he had to look at the analyst. It makes it easier for him to use the analyst as a sounding board. And finally, by reducing the activity of his other senses, it helps the patient to talk, as it helps the analyst to listen.

Admittedly, the use of the couch has certain disadvantages. Since it is designed to help the patient discover his inner psychic mechanisms, the couch produces at times a feeling of isolation, the sensation that "I am talking to myself." This is not necessarily harmful, but for certain periods of the analysis the negative aspects may outweigh the gains. Some analysts prefer a period of sitting up prior to the use of the couch, as a sort of education for analysis. Other analysts use the couch with some patients and not with others. There is no question but that the couch does stimulate fantasies in some people and thus it can become a detour from the hard road to reality and health. In such situations, as in the analysis of children, the use of the couch is not indicated.

The couch as a symbol of analysis is about as significant as the white coat for the physician. The heart of psychoanalysis is discovery of the inner world of the individual, and it is this turbulent world that the analyst is confronted with throughout the whole process. He sees the untamed, primitive world of the unconscious, the expressions of infantile desires and anger, the sick preoccupation with fantasies, the wishes to die and to kill. He listens to the patient's loneliness and hostility, struggles hour by hour with the patient's clinging to his inner tormentors — with the torturous hunger for pain as the only way of experiencing the self. He hears his patient's wistful cries for love and support and happiness. And as he sees what life has done to the patient, he focuses more and more sharply on the nature of the fractures, on the hidden strength, on the patient's wish to live and to create pleasure instead of pain for himself.

The necessity of reliving, re-experiencing, makes the psychoanalytic method of treatment different from all others. And it explains why intellectual understanding does not suffice. If this were enough, prospective psychoanalysts, after completing their studies in the classroom and the laboratory, would be qualified to practice, as is the case in other methods of treatment. Psychoanalysts, however, are required to experience analysis of their own psyche before they even begin to study the theory and technique of it. They have to experience the workings of their own unconscious before they can understand the unconscious in their patients.

The whole idea of the "unconscious" does not have much reality for any patient until his attention has been turned toward the workings of this part of his psyche. It is one thing to speak of something being "subconscious" — which customarily means preconscious, and fairly near the surface of conscious knowledge — and quite another to grasp fully the implications of the idea that all of us are only partially aware of the reasons for our actions. Usually this partial, conscious awareness is enough for rational living; sometimes it is not. Usually we make no more contact with our unconscious mind than we make with our internal organs. Few of us have full knowledge of where these organs are located, how they function, or what their purpose is — and we don't care, because there is usually no need to be aware of their existence. Similarly, we know that there is a part of the mind known as the unconscious, but as long as it doesn't bother us, we are not seriously concerned with it. To be sure, many people nowadays playfully speculate about their unconscious reasons for forgetting something, or about what made them do the very thing they meant not to do. But there are few who really understand the complicated system of the unconscious. This is due in part to the fact that the scientific discovery of the unconscious is less than a century old.

For uncountable time, "mind" has meant consciousness. Thinking and reasoning, indeed all mental life, have been considered functions of the conscious mind. The discovery of a substratum of mind with a far greater influence on human conduct than consciousness was tremendously shocking to people, and the disturbing implications of this discovery explain in part the hostility toward and fear of psychoanalysis. Although the records of mythology, of poetry, and of drama show very clearly that man has always needed to find explanations for human behavior outside the conscious mind, it is more comforting to ascribe unexplainable behavior to superhuman causes than to hidden drives within ourselves.

It is quite understandable, then, that patients come to analysis with skepticism and negative feelings, latent if not overt. They cannot confront the existence of an unknown part of the mind without some trepidation or hostility. Even after we have conceded that there is more to the psyche than is conscious or meets the eye or any of the other senses, we hesitate, quite naturally, to follow a stranger on a journey into the hitherto unknown parts of the mind.

Sooner or later, this journey leads into the formidable labyrinth called memory, one of the most intricate mazes known to man. If we knew half as much about memory as we do about the atom, we could be more effective in our analytic explorations, our educational methods, our general understanding of human behavior.

Imperfectly though we understand it, memory is one of the major theaters of analytic operation. When Freud suggested that the neurotic suffers from "forgotten memories," he indicated one of the important mechanisms of the unconscious — the human ability to put certain perceptions or sensations so far back into the memory file that they appear to be lost. We have "forgotten" the event: apparently the whole thing never happened. Short of this extreme mechanism, we usually misfile only parts of an experience or distort it enough to make it acceptable to our conscious mind.

Patients discover in analysis that "forgotten" events return to consciousness. They discover feelings or experiences of which they have not been conscious for years. And as the necessity for forgetting is removed, older feelings return. In dreams, people whom one may not have thought of for a quarter of a century or more begin to appear. Some memories return strongly and hide still more important events which are forgotten — that is, not yet recalled. Since the reliving of the past, which is basic to psychoanalysis, concerns itself mainly with the unconscious or partly conscious part of the mind, time is not relevant. Therefore, reliving past experiences does not necessarily mean talking about infancy or childhood.

A patient in analysis started each of her sessions with a prolonged silence for many months. When encouraged to say whatever came to her mind, she would answer that her mind was a blank — not a single association. This was true as far as her conscious mind was concerned, but it could not be true for the unconscious and preconscious layers of the mind, where there is always activity of some sort: feeling, certain kinds of thinking, fantasy. None of these activities had reached a state of consciousness where they could then be expressed in words and associations. A certain obstacle had been erected between the preconscious and conscious level of the mind. This impediment, which is largely beyond control of the rational mind, is called resistance. Unlike the popular meaning of the term, which is stubbornness or an unwillingness to cooperate, the psychoanalytic meaning of resistance is the inability to overcome the obstacle and make contact with the preconscious layers of the mind. The executive part of the personality, the ego, is not strong enough and is being overwhelmed by unconscious forces. Throughout the whole analytic process, resistance keeps appearing and has to be analyzed, so that the unconscious forces can be exposed to the light of conscious reason. The purpose of the resistance mechanism is to keep the infantile drives and fantasies protected. As the mechanism is analyzed, the infantile wishes become exposed, the controlling force of the personality, the ego, becomes stronger and gains more and more power over the infantile parts of the self. As Freud put it, where id was, there ego shall be.

How is the resistance taken apart, analyzed? Essentially by discovering in minute detail how it manifests itself in the relationship between analyst and patient. Once the analyst understands this, he can communicate this discovery to the patient and thereby give the patient's ego a new weapon against the infantile forces. Since the unconscious finds ever new disguises, the analyst has to remain alert throughout every moment of every analytic hour. For example, in the case of the silent patient mentioned above, the analyst noticed that whenever he went to the waiting room to ask her in, she would be smiling with embarrassment. After she entered the consultation room, the embarrassed smile would disappear and there would be prolonged silence.

This small observation proved to be crucial in uncovering one aspect of the resistance. When the analyst communicated it to the patient, she said she felt silly talking about something as trivial as this. Encouraged to censor nothing, she confessed that she had noticed lately that she was listening to the analyst's steps in the small hall between his consultation room and his waiting room. The patient went on to relate that she was amused by the slight creaking noise which the doorknob made when the analyst opened the door.

While the content of this association seemed indeed trivial, the tone of the patient's voice disclosed that she was referring to feelings highly charged with emotion. She sounded excited and extremely uncomfortable, and her fingernails were digging into her arms. The analyst assumed that behind this listening for his footsteps and the creaking of the doorknob, material was hidden that was most relevant to the resistance which produced the silence at the beginning of every hour.

He asked the patient to try to remember when she might have listened to somebody's footsteps before and been excited by the turning of a doorknob. After some associations that led to early childhood, the patient recalled with a start that she used to lie awake in her bed, waiting for her father to return from his nighttime job and enter her room. He himself had slept in this room during all the years of his night work in order not to disturb his wife, who was a light sleeper. He would come into the small hall, turn the creaking doorknob, and tiptoe into the room, where the patient — then a five-year-old girl — was waiting, pretending to sleep. He would immediately see whether she was wet, and if she was dry he would take her to the bathroom. Whether or not in handling her he inadvertently touched her genitals, the little girl found the nightly ritual a highly stimulating, early sexual experience. But this she had never admitted to herself, pretending all through the years that she was really sleeping and was not even conscious of her father's coming to her.

In this session, as the excitement over hearing the doorknob turn was analyzed, she recognized for the first time, with full force, what she had hidden from herself for over twenty years: that she had had fantasies of being her father's favorite woman and of having a sexual experience with him. The discovery of this hitherto unknown feeling in relation to the analyst's turning the doorknob is an example of what psychoanalysis calls transference. The patient was re-experiencing with the person of the analyst a very early feeling which had originally been connected with the person of the father. The significant aspect of the transference, a crucial concept which is often oversimplified, is that it enabled the patient to become conscious of a wish which had been unconscious until then. This work done by the analyst and patient is called "analyzing the resistance in the transference" and is the most characteristic aspect of the analytic treatment method.

The nature of the resistances and the state of readiness to work through them and give up infantile satisfactions determine to a high degree the length of an analysis. If one is to generalize about the length of an analysis, one would do well to use as a measure not calendar time but the analytic fifty-minute hour.

A survey undertaken in Great Britain by practicing analysts disclosed that a complete analysis averaged about eight hundred hours. Another estimate, made by the American Psychoanalytic Association, came to about seven hundred hours (for students in analytic training). On the basis of these two surveys, it would be realistic to think of seven to eight hundred hours as the probable length of a complete analysis. Since most American analysts have adopted the four-visits-a-week practice, and usually take a month's vacation, the eight hundred hours are spread out over four to five years. At twenty to thirty dollars a session — the current analytic fee among most American analysts; a fee, incidentally, which is less than many medical doctors, who see several patients per hour, charge for their time — the long duration of the average analysis makes the expense prohibitive for most people. This, of course, is one important reason why psychoanalysis as a treatment has not found the place in our society that its scientific validity deserves. It also explains why there is a continuous search for short-cut methods — for therapies that do not require so much of the patient's time and money.

The question is whether quantitative reduction does not seriously affect the effectiveness of the treatment. Most analysts would agree that twice-a-week therapy cannot be considered a full analysis. These analysts may themselves have patients whom they see twice a week, but are not attempting a full analysis with them; they have deliberately limited treatment methods and treatment goals.

What, then, is available for people who need a full analysis and cannot afford it?

There are the clinical services offered by the several analytic training institutes, where a fortunate applicant may get a full analysis for a fee commensurate with his income. Some insurance companies pay part of the expense of psychoanalysis or other forms of psychotherapy, thereby bringing them within the reach of some middle-class incomes. Those who cannot obtain such help in meeting the cost of a full analysis must have recourse to other forms of psychotherapy. These are provided by the mental hygiene services in this country, which have psychiatrists as well as other specialists: the mental hygiene clinics in many hospitals, the child guidance clinics attached to many school systems, traveling county mental hygiene units, social agencies, family casework services, and the guidance and counseling facilities in many communities, including reading clinics and pastoral counseling. While it is well to keep in mind that these vitally needed services provide nothing comparable to full analysis, it can be said that many use methods which owe much to psychoanalysis.

The layman who finds analytic fees unduly high is possibly not fully aware how much time and expense goes into the training of a properly qualified psychoanalyst. This training is if anything longer than that for any specialist in medicine or surgery, and most psychoanalysts are approaching or even past thirty before they start to earn a living from analysis. The training of an analyst has four aspects — the pre-analytic training, the analyst's personal analysis, theoretical analytic training, and supervision while in training.

The issue of pre-analytic training has been controversial from the beginning of psychoanalysis, and apparently it will continue to be for some time to come. Should the future analyst first study medicine? Or would it be more practical if he first studied psychology or related behavioral sciences and then went on to special analytic training? There have been strong cases for and against each of these points of view. They differ with the country and the educational philosophy. Freud himself consistently maintained that pre-analytic training was not significant, that only the candidate's own analysis and special analytic training mattered. However, Freud's stand failed to settle the issue of pre-analytic training. Although many people agreed with his position — as many analysts do today — there are many more practitioners who insist that medical training is important, if not essential. Both camps agree on one thing — the psychoanalyst practices psychoanalysis, not medicine. In practice both the medical and the nonmedical analyst suggest that the patient see a physician when he has physical symptoms or when organic disturbances are suspected. While controversy on the question of medical accreditation continues, the prevailing situation is roughly as follows: in the United States, the vast majority of classically trained analysts have a medical degree, whereas in Europe there is a more even division between those with a medical background and those with other credentials.

If Freud did not prevail on the question of pre-analytic training, he certainly triumphed completely on a more crucial issue — that a personal analysis be a basic requirement for the practice of psychoanalysis. Today the so-called "training analysis" is the core of psychoanalytic education.

At some point during his analysis, the student will begin to take his theoretical training. Each country and each city has its own modification of the main tenets of training. But a four-year curriculum is standard procedure in all analytic training centers. While the student is taking this curriculum, he is also beginning to learn the practice of psychoanalysis. His training institute will assign a patient to him. The student, who has by then studied the theory of psychoanalytic technique, will start to analyze his first patient, reporting weekly to one of his teachers on the course of this first analysis. The teacher, known as the supervisory analyst, is usually not the student's former training analyst.

While the candidate's training analysis is a therapeutic experience, his supervisory analysis is an educational one. A candidate who has more than one patient may have several supervisory or control analysts, and he will continue to use analysts for control and supervision for several years following his four-year course.

After the completion of a satisfactory personal training analysis, the four-year curriculum, and several years of supervision of cases, a candidate may or may not be certified by the training institute, which controls the total process. The candidate's analyst, instructors and supervisors have to agree that he can meet the requirements of the profession before he is sent out and allowed to practice on his own.

The training institutes grew out of professional associations, such as the New York Psychoanalytic Society. An accredited candidate will become a member of this group or other professional organizations, and it is this affiliation that provides the safeguard for the public, since no specialized degrees are available. The largest association of training centers for psychoanalysts is the American Psychoanalytic Association.

There are also analysts whose training antedates the formation of the best-known professional associations, and there are experienced practitioners who have obtained their training from outstanding analysts of long experience. In any case, trained and qualified analysts usually belong to professional organizations which are easily identified by membership lists. But given the requisite qualifications, there remains the individual personality of the analyst: his artistry, his talent for communicating, in short his individuality.

Two kinds of myths persist about analysts or therapists. One is that analysts' personal adjustments are notoriously poor — that they have more divorces and more maladjusted children than other people. The other is the opposite — that analysts have mastered all their emotional problems and run their lives with perfect "maturity." These myths parallel the black-and-white kind of thinking that one finds in phases of childhood about parental figures — parents are either utterly terrible or they are incredibly wonderful. Analysts have their own troubles, just as their patients do; though they have been analyzed they have not necessarily solved all their problems for all time.

What occupational generalizations could one make about analysts? It would be reasonable to assume that a good analyst, who has had some years of experience, has had to become modest in his attitude toward his patients, because he has discovered the never-ending complexity and intricacy of the human psyche. There are other by-products of having analyzed people for some time. Besides real modesty, a good analyst will have had to become a warm, alert and flexible human being with an inner readiness to understand and to care. Unless he has developed these qualities, he will not be able to follow his patients' associations, day after day, with both intuition and scientific knowledge.

People are frequently under the impression that the analyst tries to fit his patient into a fixed theoretical frame. This is a misunderstanding or an oversimplification. The theory of psychoanalysis, like all theories, is by definition a generalization. In the natural sciences, the generalizations can lead to definite laws because variables can be controlled and results predicted. But the individuality of each human being is a variable that defies all exact prediction. Since no two organisms, no two psychical structures, are alike, it is never possible accurately to duplicate experiences or to predict behavior. Absolute laws are not possible in understanding individuals. One can say, for example, that infants who are separated from a mothering figure in the first two months of life will experience feelings of deprivation. But how they will cope with this deprivation cannot be predicted. Whether they will compensate for it with increased aggression or succumb to it with massive withdrawal will require clinical observation in minute detail.

Indeed, one of the most common fallacies about psychoanalysis is the belief that it can tell us how one particular event in early life will affect character structure and even life development. How could one, for example, predict the effect of even such a major event in a child's life as the death of a parent? How was the event perceived, how much of it was recognized with full consciousness, how much was pushed into deep layers of the unconscious? At what time of the life development did this event take place? Was it at a time when the child was very attached to the parent and might experience a feeling of desertion? Or was it at a phase when the child unconsciously wished for the parent's death? Would the event lend credence to the child's fantasies and strengthen the illusion that our secret wishes can indeed affect reality? Might it increase irrational feelings of guilt? What would be the feelings of the surviving parent and how much would the child identify with this parent? How much would it change his position in relation to brothers or sisters? How did the event change the economic or cultural life of the family and the child?

These are only a few of the many variables which would determine how such an event might affect the development of one individual. Without understanding what a given event has meant to an individual *on all levels of his personality*, one could not possibly make any assumptions or predictions about its effects.

There is no short cut to real understanding of a human being. It requires the slow and patient analysis of all parts

of the personality, with utmost awareness of the uniqueness of each individual's differences from other individuals. Because of this the analyst cannot possibly succeed
unless he himself is free of rigidity in thinking and un-
encumbered by authoritarian attitudes. The first-rate
practitioner cannot be arrogant or make himself out to
be a magician who can read another person's mind. He
will have had to develop a healthy respect for the intrac-
tability of many character structures. He will have had to
develop a certain simplicity from the compassionate neutrality that is one of the necessary attitudes in this work.
He will have to possess a good deal of warmth and some
humor in order to maintain the necessary balance in the
face of so much tension in his patients, hour after hour.
These qualities are not reflected in the framed diplomas
of academic degrees or in the number of professional
affiliations listed in membership directories, but they are
what the patient should look for in his search for the right
therapist.

Extracts from the Writings
of Sigmund Freud

———•———

I am not really a man of science. . . . I am nothing but by temperament a conquistador — an adventurer . . . with the curiosity, the boldness, and the tenacity that belongs to that type of being.

A man who has been the indisputable favorite of his mother keeps for life the feeling of a conqueror — that confidence of success that often induces real success.

Why should analyzed people be altogether better than others? Analysis makes for *unity,* but not necessarily for *goodness.* . . . I think that too heavy a burden is laid on analysis when one asks of it that it should be able to realize every precious ideal.

Geniuses are unbearable people. You have only to ask my family to learn how easy I am to live with, so I certainly cannot be a genius.

The great question . . . which I have not been able to

answer, despite my thirty years of research into the feminine soul, is "What does a woman want?"

My life has been aimed at one goal only: to infer or to guess how the mental apparatus is constructed and what forces interplay and counteract there.

They may abuse my doctrines by day, but I am sure they dream of them at night.

Imaginative writers are valuable colleagues [of the psychoanalyst], and their testimony is to be rated very highly, because they have a way of knowing many of the things between heaven and earth which are not dreamed of in our philosophy.

In the expressions of the psyche, there is nothing trifling, nothing arbitrary and lawless.

I have to be somewhat miserable in order to write well.

Happiness is the deferred fulfillment of a prehistoric wish. That is why wealth brings so little happiness; money is not an infantile wish.

[The goal of psychoanalysis is] to substitute for neurotic misery ordinary human unhappiness.

It seems to be my fate to discover only the obvious: that children have sexual feelings, which every nursemaid knows; and that night dreams are just as much wish-fulfillment as daydreams.

Freud and Jung

GERALD SYKES

———•———

I

THE dispassionate calm of scientists is traditional. I too believed in it — until I began to look at scientists scientifically. As a novelist and literary critic, I had taken an amateur's interest in psychology, written a few articles about it, and finally signed a contract with a publisher to do a book about it. Thereafter I met psychologists by the dozen and made the discovery that they were every bit as emotional as anybody else.

They are especially emotional on one subject — "that thing about Freud and Jung," as one of my literary friends had called it while prudently warning me against my project. Not since boyhood quarrels in Kentucky about the relative merits of Lee and Grant had I encountered such polemical intensity. To some people Freud was personally responsible for most teen-age delinquency; to others Jung was so vague and mystical as to be absolutely unreadable. To some Freud stood for an outdated positivism that now impeded any clear thinking about our real problem; to others Jung was anti-Semitic and pro-Nazi.

After years of research I have come to the conclusion that there is no truth in any of these accusations. I believe they are all rationalizations, and rationalizations to which many others who are not professional psychologists are also addicted. I believe that Freud and Jung stand for opposing sides of the human mind, that their dialogue is central enough to invite comparison with characters in Greek tragedy, and that when we denounce one or the other we merely reveal our incapacity to confront an unknown portion of ourselves. None of these accusations would stand up after close scrutiny of the lives and work of the men in question; all of these accusations have been publicly exploded long ago. Yet they persist. Why? Because people want scapegoats for their own intellectual laziness and their own spiritual cowardice.

But there is more to it than that. Psychology establishes such an intimate and powerful hold upon its students that once allegiance has been given to any school — and each of us must begin with a single school, the one to which we are naturally drawn — a complete change of intellectual habits is required before we can even become aware of other schools. And then our first reaction is bound to be one of pain and distaste. The progress from psychology to comparative psychology — a progress that many people are going to have to make, unless there is to be a return to the rancor of the religious wars, with modern demagogic complications — is always hard.

A brief preliminary examination of the lives and works of Freud and Jung will show why this is so. Fortunately, they are so eloquent, they embody so dramatically two opposite sides of the mind and of contemporary experience, that they turn dry elucidation into good theater. Together they form one of psychology's most far-reaching debates — and an excellent introduction to problems that sooner or later each of us must face.

The name of Freud is usually associated with what has

been called the sexual revolution. Actually, that event began long before he did his work. Historically, it can be traced to the industrial revolution. It began in fact as a protest against the antihuman tendencies of that event and its poetic forefathers were Blake and Whitman.

This lyric movement has since had to face the counterattack of tradition and is intellectually on the defensive today, but it still continues as a protest. The typical sexual rebel believes in sex with religious fervor. His rebellion seems to vary according to his sense of a lost spiritual heritage, and when he feels himself utterly disowned of a tradition that he can accept — cut off, so to speak, with a library card — he can become a satyr. Orgasm is his substitute for feeling. This is a development that Whitman could not have foreseen. The effect of industrialism upon love has been so drastic as to make a great many people demand physical gratification in lieu of every other amorous reward. It has generated an unprecedented mass fear of impotence. In a world of steel and asphalt, sex takes over certain aspects of the divine.

There has probably been more moralizing on this than on any other phase of twentieth-century life. Most of this moralizing has been beside the point because it has failed to take into account just these historical crosscurrents. We could not want a better example of why a sound understanding of psychology must precede a sound understanding of morals.

Freud's ideas on this complex and highly controversial subject are often misunderstood. In effect he wrote that sex is impersonal, nature blindly concerned with her own propagation, and that if we attach the wrong emotions to our part of the process, if we remain ignorant of the unconscious forces that are the principal determinants of our behavior, we become ill both in mind and in body. Health requires that we be aware of these unconscious forces, which originate in early childhood, so that we can sublimate them in socially acceptable tasks.

It is a stern doctrine, but it has been confused with moral laxity because it calls for close examination of a subject that is generally regarded as unsavory. If it means a release from inhibitions, it also imposes — after a trying experimental period which is the real reason why traditional moralists fear it — still stricter standards in their place. If it takes a deterministic attitude toward previous morality, it goes on to demand another which is much more difficult to observe.

Sex seems to have been the road Freud had not taken, the life he had not lived. As a family man his life was extremely correct. One biographer states flatly that he never had any sexual experience outside marriage. This is unprovable but significant. It suggests that the man whose name more than any other is linked with broad sexual knowledge had little of it through personal experience.

No spinster, certainly, was ever more aware of every erotic nuance. Sex was his poetry. Together with his extraordinary talents, this was what made him so persuasive. But he was also aided by the fact that he was Jewish. As in the case of Marx, his scientific achievements were part of the expansion of a gifted, ancient, persecuted people which had only recently emerged from the ghetto. This people had an extraordinary insight into the evils of a decadent Christianity, an insight, born of a vigorous intellectual tradition and a long experience of injustice, that lent itself especially to reductive analysis. Marx had reduced the evils of the political economy to the profit motive and predicted that under socialism the state would wither away. Freud reduced the evils of the inner life to misunderstanding of the erotic instinct and predicted that after psychoanalysis the mind would become healthy. Each put his finger on a weak spot in an enemy position that he was supremely qualified, not only through his private talents but through his background, to expose to the world.

It has now become apparent that both these great insights suffered from oversimplification. Men's disillusionment with Marxism came earlier and on a larger scale. This has led often to a denial of its values. Freudianism had no Russia to work on, and by its nature it is less on parade, but disillusionment with it continues and may diminish its perceptions for those who need them most. It is nevertheless a very powerful movement, especially among those urbanized people who have felt the attack of industrialism upon their instincts. It is particularly strong among city dwellers in the United States today, and for just this reason. Our city dwellers have usually become aware of their psychological problems through sexual and economic frustrations. A treatment, therefore, which may release them from erotic and aggressive inhibitions has the dramatic appeal of a psychic appendectomy, promising not only health but happiness and prosperity as well. It is the sort of down-to-earth treatment that makes sense in a busy marketplace.

So Freud's therapy is definitely related to the industrial revolution. This will become clearer when it is compared to the therapy of Jung, who came forward a little later to call attention to those aspects of the inner life that had been relatively unaffected — or affected in another way — by technology. In response to the needs of a suffering and confused humanity, our period has produced not only the specifically *contemporary* psychology of Freud but the relatively *timeless* psychology of Jung. The two unite in a dialogue admirably suited to comparison. *Not,* however, to controversy. I hope it will be clear why a partisan attitude in this debate is especially barren.

Offhand the timeless quality of Jung's psychology would seem fatal to it. Certainly it does not appear to equip it for survival in an age which daily grows more industrial, more political, more warlike. His psychology is somewhat like a Platonic academy in the midst of a radioactive battlefield. It differs also from our socially useful academies in its open doubt of the intellect, at least the intellect as characteristically employed today. Far from admiring the typical mentality of our urban culture, Jung mistrusts it.

Jung was a Swiss, and his psychology reflects the desire of his people — and of others like them — to live an orderly, traditional life in an era of violent change. In contrast to most Jews — who are born inescapably into turmoil — most Swiss try to stay out of it. Jung cannot be "explained" by his Swissness, any more than Freud can be "explained" by his Jewishness, but in each, beneath the accomplishments of a truly international mind, resides an impersonal element, identifiable with his people, which helps greatly in the exposition of modern psychology because it polarizes modern social experience.

Jung's silent invocations are rural and classic rather than urban and modern. Thus his work would seem to be as anachronistic, as unreal, as cultish as his opponents have described it, if there were not always classic problems among the most contemporary and if a truly modern consciousness did not also have to contend with them.

It is Jung's anachronism, in fact, his seeming irrelevance, that constitutes finally his greatest strength — at least for those who, as youth deserts them, begin to realize that not all their problems turn on childhood influences or the encroachment of civilization upon instinct; that there are other problems equally pressing and as old as the hills.

But to understand the origin of Jung's ideas it is necessary, as it is with Freud, to know a few facts about his life. He was born in 1875 in Switzerland, the son of a Protestant clergyman, and for our time had a life of privileged tranquillity. He was a paleontologist and classical scholar as well as a psychologist, traveled widely throughout the world, and lived, until his death in 1961, on the shores of Lake Zurich.

From these bare facts emerge four important considerations:

First, Jung was born into a period later than Freud's, when natural science felt somewhat less confidence in its powers to explain all or almost all of life. Jung was therefore encouraged to devote some of his scientific energy to philosophical problems that Freud had expressly excluded from the purview of psychoanalysis.

Second, Jung had a temperament that was expansive rather than reductive and that led him in time to rebel against what he called Freud's "nothing but" analysis. Gifted with a robust constitution and a robust attitude toward nature — until shortly before his death he vacationed periodically in a remote, electricity-less, servantless house that he built himself — he did not make a poetry of the biological, but of the divine.

Third, he became scientifically as much interested in religion as Freud had been in Eros, and discovered within himself a similar pioneering genius in its study.

Fourth, although he was born into less conflict with society than Freud, their roles have been reversed since the positivism championed by Freud has become a new orthodoxy. Now it is Jung who is at greater variance with the intellectual mores of his day.

Freud believed that the mind of man could be explained, if one persisted long enough, in terms of his *immediate environment*. Jung believed that one can only begin to understand it by going back to all of the many factors which entered into its making, which lead in every case to the *remote past*. It can be demonstrated, he says, that we are commonly possessed by archetypes as old as the race itself. Such a perspective will dismay the quick, pragmatic, modern temper, which can only feel equal to its problems by jettisoning most of the past, but such a perspective, Jung says, is the only way to truth and health. Once Christianity was overturned, modern man had to face all the internal demons that the Church had kept at bay for him. The way to rebuild our lives is to relax the will, stop being merely contemporary, and seek harmony with nature. Our troubles are erotic, especially when we are young, but they are many other things as well, and the first step in dealing with them is to see them in historical scale. Only in so doing will we find a durable sense of purpose, and we need a sense of purpose quite as much as we need biological fulfillment.

The roots of character are not all here and now, and even the most elaborate autobiographical search will not uncover more than a few of them. Society is as sick as Freud says it is, but we need not be — if we are willing and able to become what we innately are.

Such a restatement of their positions is fair to neither Freud nor Jung. But even these glimpses will indicate the nature and sources of their conflict. And if we try to understand it, we see that it is as human, as foreordained, as meaningful as the conflict between two heroic characters in a Greek tragedy. These men are not only historic personages, they are also parts of ourselves and they enact a play that goes on daily in our own minds. We all have to live in the vigorously contemporary world of Freud, and we all have to live in the archetypal world of Jung. We have to be effective; we also have to be in harmony with nature. To do both of these things at the same time is as difficult as any demand we can make upon ourselves. Our natural tendency, therefore, will be to take sides with one of them against the other, but if we do we shall neither enjoy their drama properly nor make the best use of it. This will be still more evident when we continue their dialogue briefly into the subject of religion.

Offhand it would seem that Freud had no use at all for religion. He traced its origin to the small child's helplessness before the outer world and to its dependence on its parents. He rejected religion specifically as an immaturity and an illusion, an inability to stand on one's own feet. He said, "Science is not an illusion. But it would be an illusion to suppose that we can get anywhere else what it cannot give us." To an American friend he wrote: "To me the moral has always appeared as self-evident." In other words, he took morality for granted and reasoned that if he could get along without religion, why couldn't other men? In this, I believe it can be demonstrated, he drew upon the *unconscious religion* concealed in his scientific credo, upon the unanalyzed faith that he got from his laboratory training.

"Unconscious religion" is a phrase used more and more today. Anti-communists use it to explain communists —

along with such words as "fanaticism," "auto-da-fé," and "grand inquisitors." Few intellectuals apply it, however, to themselves; they prefer to think that they have rationally transcended all religious motivations, which at least will never trouble *them*. In other words, the repressions of the nineteenth century have been reversed in the twentieth. They are no longer sexual, they are religious. To deny the many-sided urge toward erotic gratification would now correctly be considered absurd. No absurdity, however, is found in a denial of the urge toward purpose, toward symbolism, toward the necessary ingredients of the will to go on. This blind spot is one of the less fortunate of Freud's legacies.

Actually, however, without knowing it, he himself made important contributions to religious thought. Three of his most familiar concepts will illustrate what I mean. The first he borrowed from Havelock Ellis and extended. *Narcissism* is a deeply imaginative attempt to deal with the problem of evil. The inescapability of self could hardly be better symbolized than by this amazingly astute reference to the self-love that must follow us wherever we go. It is a splendid instance of the biological honesty that is indispensable to true spirituality.

His *superego* likewise provides a valuable distinction between morbid self-criticism and the healthy self-criticism needed for making truly responsible moral decisions. History is full of weaklings terrorized and crippled by power-seeking priesthoods through perverted appeals to conscience. Every ecclesiastical reformation has been in part a purge of a corrupt misuse of the sense of guilt. And this is no longer solely a religious problem but now an acute political one.

Finally, Freud's *death instinct*, when juxtaposed to its

opposite, the life instinct, or Eros in its fullest sense, is seen as exactly the kind of symbolic tool that Freud's realism was brilliantly equipped to add to our thought. No one can fail to learn much about his own psychological rhythms by observing the alternations of these two opposing instincts within himself. And this kind of systole-diastole insight can lead to a philosophic balance that is not far from the idea expressed by Dante in *The Divine Comedy.* "In His will is our peace." There was much unconscious religion indeed in Freud.

There is in everyone. We are all full of it, according to our temperaments, and we shall be happier — or better able to choose a tragedy worthy of us — if we become aware of it. This was the discovery of Jung, which he announced at a time when such a point of view had become scientifically scandalous. He said he had found proof of the therapeutic effect of genuine religious experience — of the role played by faith, not in immaturity but in maturity. He made an issue of it. He announced cures. He spoke of highly educated patients who had been freed of their anxiety when they discovered the limits of reason, when they rediscovered symbolism and mystery. He wrote: "I take carefully into account the symbols produced by the unconscious mind. They are the only things able to convince the critical mind of modern people. . . . The thing that cures a neurosis must be as convincing as the neurosis; and since the latter is only too real, the helpful experience must be of equal reality."

Jung, however, was by no means a naïve, uncritical enthusiast of the religious life. He did not point the way to easy faith. Like William James, he saw religion as a force subject to the laws of the mind which could lead either to good or to evil. He explored the different responses to it in different types of men. In the face of Freud's attempt to dismiss it as an illusion, he drove home his empirical discovery that it was a fact, a fact that could not be conveniently traced to the nursery and forgotten. In this matter it seems to me that he was right, and that Freud's own life and work prove his point.

On the other hand, how many people can afford to live in the epicurean detachment that Jung's prescription implies? This is a question raised by Jung's opponents. Economically, the whole trend of modern life is against his attitude, which is bound to become rarer and rarer. And would not such detachment lead to a washing of the hands, in the elegant manner of Pontius Pilate, of the urgent political and social problems that must be faced if the commonwealth is to advance in decency and justice? A civic stance acquired in lucky, war-free isolation is apt to be irrelevant. Jung's programmatic introversion is an anachronistic luxury that could only be afforded in times free of unrest, times not at all like our own. To cling to it now is mere nostalgia. Such critcism seems to be the core of the opposition to Jung.

The core of the opposition to Freud seems to be that people are not as simple as he saw them, but many rootless moderns have embraced his oversimplifications with a monomaniacal devotion that is now in the process of dehumanizing them. Our urbanized culture is producing overpragmatic monsters whose cynical first question is "What's in it for me?" Freud's reality principle, therefore, except for some overimpressionable and overprivileged intellectuals, is only so many words. In practice, together with the ethical lobotomy that usually accompanies it, it has led to a deplorable opportunism that will soon lay waste, and often in the name of decency and justice, whatever remains of the moral foundations of society.

There is plainly an element of truth in both these oppositions. Both of them are emotional, both of them are exaggerated, but in each there is enough basis in fact to have made it possible to rationalize them into full-scale hatreds. That is why most people's attitude toward psychology's most heated debate remains bitterly one-sided. It is so much easier to emotionalize our inner conflicts. It is so hard to live with them, to see their pros and cons, to weave them patiently together.

How to weave them together? That, together with the interweaving of still other theories by still other men, is *the* problem of comparative psychology. It calls for a union of tension and relaxation. The thought of Freud is essentially tense. It is a product of struggle, of a life that was not permitted much calm. There is a sense of urgency about it, and its goal is less happiness than effectiveness. It is far more revolutionary than its opposite, at least in social impact. It is more startling, more dramatic, more in the idiom of our century. It prepares men for survival in a time of general shipwreck. It is above all practical: one is called upon to eliminate one's irrational impulses, by becoming aware of their childhood origins, and to strengthen the conscious mind. It is only in this way that one can accomplish anything worthwhile, right any wrongs, eradicate any ignorance, make an impression on an indifferent universe.

The thought of Jung is esentially relaxed. It is addressed to those who wish to fulfill their inner potentialities even in an era of drastic change. It refuses to get alarmed over financial and political crises. It is a product of relative tranquillity. It puts a minimum of emphasis on social adaptation, which it regards as a necessary first hurdle rather than as a lifework, and a maximum of emphasis on internal development. It is especially addressed to people over thirty-five, and it finds scientific sanction for love of fate and attunement to nature.

To weave together such entirely different attitudes may be necessary for the creation of a truly successful human being, but it will obviously be an infrequent accomplishment. No wonder most people would rather quarrel ignorantly about it.

But there is another reason why Freud and Jung continue to provide a convenient battleground for quickly stirred emotions. They not only embody some of our most central dramas; in their combination of elderliness and wisdom they are both father figures par excellence. At heart we are childish, we want to confer magic on imaginary papas.

An unrecorded part of history is the expropriation of magic. The priest took it away from the medicine man, and the medical man took it away from the priest. For most of us the mind doctor does not have as much of it as the body doctor, because he does not scare us as much. But for those who get caught up in psychological problems this is not true. The mind doctor turns into the most awesome figure of all, especially when he is a theorist, a name. We shall be happier, I think — or at least more ourselves — when we stop conferring magic on anyone. We are born partisan. We do not have to remain so.

Jung's manner is strikingly unlike Freud's gloom. Jung is hearty; for him the forces of the unconscious are not always dark and primitive; they can also, if understood, liberate and dignify. Dreams are not always infantile wish-fulfillments; they can also be adultly teleological, i.e., work toward a cure and a release of creative power. And he does not consider religion an "illusion" if it succeeds, as he reports it has succeeded with many of his patients, in healing their neuroses: "The thing that cures a neurosis must be as convincing as the neurosis; and since the latter is only too real, the helpful experience must be of equal reality. But what is the difference between a real illusion and a healing religious experience? It is merely a difference in words. You can say, for instance, that life is a disease with a very bad prognosis, it lingers on for years to end in death; or that normality is a generally prevailing constitutional defect; or that man is an animal with a fatally overgrown brain. This kind of thinking is the prerogative of habitual grumblers with bad digestions. Nobody can know what the ultimate things are. We must, therefore, take them as we experience them. And if such experience helps to make our life healthier, more beautiful, more complete and more satisfactory to yourself and to those you love, you may safely say: 'This was the grace of God.' "

This will hearten the tender-minded and dismay the tough-minded, to whom it will seem to endorse, too unguardedly, just those obscurantist and regressive forces which are only too ready to kite such an appeal into a blank check for any kind of religiosity and, by extension, any kind of political exploitation of religiosity. Progressives find that it descends to polite demagogy and attempts to ingratiate its author with the more conservative members of the Yale University audience which first heard it. Headlined, it might read: SCIENTIST OKAYS GOD. Even by private standards, with no reference to possible abuses or distortions, such a statement suggests that one's inner voice is more reliable than anyone but a well-disciplined mystic, who would hardly need such encouragement, has any right to expect. It reiterates the confidence of the "inner-directed." Are not the insane asylums full of those who imagine they have a direct pipeline to the Holy Ghost? Do not the milder cases of religious certitude join our army of sensitive ineffectuals, who have shrunk away from the healthy give-and-take of the marketplace into one elegant retreat or another? Is it not reckless to encourage them in their soul-searching, their art-major mandalas? All this seems like a decadent form of upper-class Protestantism when put next to the stern counsels of Freud, who warns specifically against such immature self-deceptions. Such, at least, has been some of the response to it.

Adler's criterion of "social interest" would also make short work of such a self-appointed search for "private meaning." More gently than Freud, but with equal firmness, he would point out that each of us must meet the test of what we do "when confronted by the unavoidable problems of humanity." If we retreat into purely decorative dilettantism we cannot lay claim to the possession of great souls. If much has been given us, then we have failed all the more lamentably. We may indeed be the worst failures, of whom he writes that "no one else is benefited by the achievement of their aims, and their interest stops short at their own persons."

It soon becomes apparent that three kinds of ethics are ensnarled here, and ensnarled so humanly that the capacity to think clearly about them is far more difficult than professionals will admit. The first is the insistence on grim truth-seeking of Freud, the second the insistence on friendly teamwork of Adler, the third the insistence on personal development of Jung. Each of them is so heavily loaded, in the context of our own lives, with our own preoccupations — usually unconscious ancestral bequests and therefore all the more explosive — that when we attempt to discuss them we are really painting our family tree. Moreover, each of these men was exceptionally gifted, and shaped his thoughts with exceptional skill — with the special cunning that comes to a strong one-sided mind when it is out to prove that it alone is right. (I overlook their more modest disclaimers as mere tricks of the trade, to beguile the unwary.) Each of these men spoke from his own portion of the unconscious more persuasively than when he spoke from his intelligence. Which is one more reason why they are best understood when seen as myth-makers, not scientists.

To return to Jung, his reply to Freud and Adler has been clear. He has said that he encounters many patients who respond best to a Freudian analysis, many patients who respond best to an Adlerian analysis, and still others, usually in middle age, who "are suffering from no clinically definable neurosis, but from the senselessness and emptiness of their lives." This, he thinks, "can well be described as the general neurosis of our time," and has led to his distinction between the "personal unconscious," that Malebolge of primitive aggressions and timorous

repressions, and the "collective unconscious," the potential
Paradiso which contains within it the seeds of rebirth that
can conquer emptiness and replace it with purpose. He
finds the theories of Freud, even in their later, revised
form, too simple. Man is not only a social creature, he
says in effect, and not only a hard-pressed mediator between Eros and Thanatos. He also has a life of his own,
and it can be a happy one.

In a sense Jung was a more practical psychologist than
the other two. He used his science to achieve personal
serenity. Adler's triumph was brief. Freud certainly enjoyed the excitement of his great discoveries and the professional satisfaction of being put on Darwin's level, but
the whole tenor of his work suggests a grave personal dis-
appointment, even among the lineaments of gratified
ambition. His heroic sublimation did not bring the joy
that his name may have promised him in boyhood. But
Jung has been *happy*. No one can read his works without
feeling his active enjoyment of life. He has achieved a
harmony with nature that seems almost classical. It has
not commended him to our crisis-ridden intellectuals. He
has been called bourgeois. His style has been described as
Brahmsian. Existentialists protest that he exudes the
reek of pre-1914 euphoria. It is plain that he is not in the
modern temper, which though nominally anti-Christian
seems to demand of its spiritual heroes an Agony in the
Garden and a Crucifixion — or at least a very painful
compulsion neurosis such as was suffered by those Christ-
obsessed flagellants Kierkegaard, Nietzsche, Dostoevski,
van Gogh. The bucolic contentment of Jung hardly com-
mends him for martyrdom, and it is martyrs that we — or
at least a respected group of moralists among us — demand these days. The obscure sexual difficulties of Freud,

as well as his cancer and his rescue in extreme old age from a brutal soldiery, are more to the taste of a generation that under the guidance of Albert Camus has made a hero of Sisyphus. (Adler does not count for much with that generation, which appears to regard him as a Foolish Virgin.)

The real reason why this generation is anti-Jung is that he does not help them in their drive for a success that might, they hope, compensate them for their unhappiness. Jung actually encourages the pleasure principle by his endorsement of a leisurely Goethean search for metaphysical values, by his hospitality to Vedanta, Taoism and Zen, by his scholarly research in Gnosticism and alchemy, by his speculations on the "archetypes," on synchronicity, on the psychoid, in short by learned investigations that would require years of contemplation and perhaps a private income. He writes as if there were no hurry at all — for a generation continually rediscovering that it has "so little time." Olympian methods of this nature are not suited to those who refuse to be students all their lives, who feel they must make their mark, and certainly their livelihood, now or never. For such down-to-earth souls the Freudian ban on the pleasure principle and its early puritan replacement by the reality principle are distinctly preferable. We only live once, and even if we *have* made our mark, we have to go on making it again and again. It is all very well to play down success — *if* you have it. Otherwise you are ignored, and after a while the public's attitude toward you becomes your own. Jung offers a nice consolation prize for the losers, something like hothouse gardening in the wintertime. He has nothing to say to those who want to win. Such charges have been made repeatedly against him.

Our realistic belief in success, success repeatedly re-established in the press and daily proclaimed by possessions, provides the core of much opposition to Jung. Another source is the desire to communicate idiomatically with one's contemporaries. Jung appears to be advocating a new brand of other-worldliness. Such is not the case. Actually Jung advocates success here and now, but of an unpopular kind: private, unrecognized, estranging success; success that means, unless one is well cushioned against the disapproval of the populace, failure and poverty. His ideas are not easily apprehended by a mind conditioned by ambition or journalism. They invite, in fact, the repudiation they so frequently encounter, and sometimes not merely because of their nature, but because of the almost perverse and provocative way their author has phrased them. The quotation from his Yale lectures will have indicated how he enjoyed, safe in his privileged coign of vantage, violating the intellectual tabus of more exposed scholars. His works abound in such prankish ambiguities, one of which, about Hitler, was notoriously infelicitous. But it is the unpopular substance of his ideas that creates most of his enemies. Numerically there is a smaller but more important resistance among those who are greatly stimulated by his thought but who, since they want to communicate with a contemporary audience which demands that ideas be given a flesh-and-blood reality such as his do not have, are forced to realize that these, like his archetypes, must be translated into the language of our day. It is a tribute to his enormous fertility of concept, a fertility that was most certainly helped by his nation's aloofness from struggle.

Jung does not conceal his mistrust of the unaided ego, that cornerstone of Freud's fortress against darkness and regression. Even before Freud came along, an ego psychology was helping to strengthen the West by increasing its technical skills and redoubling its Faustian will to control the forces of nature; but now, Jung suggests, this exploitative mentality, though the East is at present feverishly trying to imitate it, has reached the point of diminishing personal returns. He therefore finds reasons to respect — though not to copy — the psychological procedures of an earlier East which is on the defensive today even in Asia. Such procedures, which seek to reinforce the ego with unused powers in the mind, increase our perspective on individual fulfillment here and now. They may not advance our technical effectiveness in a marketplace that requires sedulous adjustment to its frenzied competition, but they may help to make life worth living.

Indirectly Joseph Campbell described Freud's position when he wrote in *The Hero with a Thousand Faces:* "Modern literature is devoted, in great measure, to a courageous, open-eyed observation of the sickeningly broken figurations that abound before us, around us, and within. . . . And there is no make-believe about heaven, future bliss, and compensation. . . . In comparison with all this, our little stories of achievement seem pitiful. . . . Hence we are not disposed to assign to comedy the high rank of tragedy." Indirectly Campbell described Jung's position when he wrote: "The happy ending of the fairy tale, the myth, and the divine comedy of the soul, is to be read, not as a contradiction, but as a transcendence of the universal tragedy of man. The objective world remains what it was, but, because of a shift in emphasis within the subject, is beheld as though transformed. Where formerly life and death contended, now enduring being is

FREUD AND JUNG · 93

made manifest. . . . The dreadful mutilations are then seen as shadows, only, of an immanent, imperishable eternity; time yields to glory; and the world sings with the prodigious, angelic, but perhaps finally monotonous, siren music of the spheres."

The distinguishing feature of Jung's psychology, as we have noted, is the "collective unconscious," which he says takes us out of our ego preoccupations, reaches back to remotest antiquity, and contains the potentials of health and integration. To clarify the "personal unconscious," as Freud does, is not enough, Jung says, but must be continued into the spontaneous, archetypal symbolism that unites all men and offers transcendence of the more banal and frustrative portions of existence. Understood and used intelligently, this symbolism can fill the spiritual vacuum that is modern man's birthright. A tasteful preference for tragedy can be a safe academic formula, rather than a confrontation of both disaster *and* glory. Tragedy will come inevitably wherever there is life, but as a concept it means nothing unless it follows a conscious struggle against it in its frequently neurotic forms. Archetypal symbolism contains the seeds of faith, but does not lead to easy serenity — rather to a lifelong, controversial value-search that tragically estranges the individual from society and resembles existentialism in its trials. The new school of existential analysis that has come into being has much in common with Jung's mistrust of a lucrative, ego-dominated "mind-body split."

Such reasoning will not mean much to most people who only want to think of psychology when they suffer from some serious and elusive disorder. It also offends the practical nature of most Americans because it does not seem to apply to their everyday problems, which, when psychiatric in origin, can be dealt with by a licensed psychiatrist. Groundlings of this sort are apt to think of Jung, when they think of him at all, as addicted to la-di-da introspection, which, at first glance, is all his psychology seems to be. The devotion of his prodigious scholarship and insight to such remote matters as faith, not to mention the Gnostics and the alchemists, at a time when our psychiatry is unable to cope with such immediate matters as divorce, alcoholism, sexual deviations, delinquency, immaturity and escapism, appears to be nothing but another escapism.

Only an uninformed reading will find it so. Actually, as a psychiatrist with enormous clinical experience, Jung knows very well what our everyday problems are; his books deal with them continually. His later works, for example, throw much new light on our latest social problems, the origin of wars, and what caused the atomic physicists to create the instrument that makes us all uneasy. Readers are still put off, however, by his seemingly oblivious manner, which grandly overlooks prevailing economic and biological orientations and coins a private language. Examination also discovers that he has not a few blind spots, can antagonize both the religious and the antireligious, attracts a cult of irresponsible devotees, can be rather insensitive on matters of literature and art, and has taken a position that must be termed esoteric. Upon closer examination, his esotericism seems deliberate — and farsighted.

Politically, he is neither the obscurantist nor the reactionary that he has been called, but he does *not* have faith in the masses. (Neither did Freud.) He believes that Western man is possessed by unconscious forces that have "robbed him of all free will." (Will, incidentally, he de-

fines as the "sum of psychic energy disposable to consciousness," which seems an excellent example of the
manner in which an ancient philosophic issue can be
clarified by a psychologist. If you are not free, it is because your mind is still relatively "primitive." If you wish
to be free, the way to it is through a new kind of "culture
and moral education.") "And this state of unconscious
possession will go on until we . . . become scared of
our god-almightiness. Such a change can only begin with
individuals, for the masses are blind brutes, as we know
to our cost. It seems to me of some importance, therefore,
that a few individuals, or people individually, should begin to understand that there are contents which do not
belong to the ego-personality but must be ascribed to a
psychic non-ego."

Modern man, he says, has lost faith in all ready-made
symbols, but he cannot be healed by the reduction of his
ailments to any single cause, however helpful it may seem
at first. To become healthy and free, man must draw upon
mental resources which come from "a psychic non-ego"
that unites him to other men and to nature. This seems
dubious to those bound by medical charts and newspaper
statistics and the shopkeepers' trust in immediate tangible
success, but is none the less real. To be of lasting use,
psychiatry should aid in building a bridge to the new, un-
tried faith that we must find for ourselves if we are not
to be destroyed by our ignorance of the true dynamics of
the psyche, which are far subtler — both more destructive and more regenerative — than Freud presents them
in a tidy meccano-like system.

Since the correction of our ignorance would require a
long period of humble study and personal dislocation, it
is not difficult to see why few undertake it. To be truly

effective, Jung's therapy means many more years of tough self-discipline than Freud's, because it calls for both a Freudian adjustment and a Jungian break with accepted social goals. Thus nothing is so understandable as the opposition of practical folk, who are more subject to the objective psyche's demons than their daily tasks will allow them to admit. When they enlist psychiatry they want a patchwork job. Meanwhile we go on producing "hollow men" who will never be able to give us the leadership we need. Nearly all Jungian patients are timid introverts seeking unnoticed secession.

Actually, there can be no "comic" transcendence of tragedy except in exceptional moments preceded and followed by suffering. There is not so much difference between Freud and Jung on this point as there seems to be, though Jung counsels a greater trust in the helpful processes in nature. Time exaggerated the difference of the two men on this issue. Freud reacted against the old arrogance of religion — which he had keenly felt in Austria — when he dismissed it as an illusion. Jung reacted against the new arrogance of science — which he had keenly felt, somewhat later, in Switzerland — when he said that under certain circumstances religion could be healthy.

He was also less identified with a strictly medical point of view than Freud. He had begun his career as a classical scholar before studying medicine, and his continuing closeness to the soil increased his detachment about his profession. "Whoever is rooted in the soil endures." Compared with Freud's equally bannerlike "Men are strong so long as they represent a strong idea," this suggests an attitude that we shall be getting soon from one of our novelists. "Remoteness from the unconscious, and therefore

from the determining influence of history, means an up-
rooted state. This is the danger . . . confronting every
individual who through one-sidedness in any kind of ism
loses his relation to the dark, maternal, earthly origin of
his being." It is one of Jung's leading ideas, and it is also
one of D. H. Lawrence's. It goes with the genial, relaxed
therapy that Jung seems to have practiced. One of his
favorite maxims is the Latin form of "Nature heals, the
physician only treats." It also suggests a more historical
attitude toward the unconscious than was possible to the
more harassed, more dramatic Freud — a difference that
can be traced to their religious backgrounds. In addition,
it may explain why Jung was not able to accept Freud's
original emphasis on sex.

Freud genuinely believed that Jung was guilty of ex-
pediency or puritanism when he wished, as Freud put it,
to "soft-pedal" sex. What Freud could not realize was that
his own emphasis on sex as a factor in psychopathology
was in part a consequence of his struggle with puritanism;
or that to Jung, who was much less of a puritan than he,
sexual disorders could at times be merely symptomatic of
still larger disturbances — disturbances which originated
in an uprooting, both physical and spiritual, of which the
patient was still less aware than of his erotic misfortunes.
Freud believed, because his own career had been mostly
limited to city laboratories and city clinics and city neuroses, that Jung wished to play safe. Actually, it would
have been more expedient at that time — 1912 — for
Jung to soft-pedal his differences with Freud and not to
insist upon his own interpretations. But Jung had to express his own relationship to nature, and Freud had to
express his, and so their rupture occurred. It was a great
shock to both of them. That much is made clear by the

amount each has written about it. But it was also a stimulant, it put them on their mettle, and each continued to influence the other — at a distance. So much the better for us: in their imperfect retinas is our vision.

Nevertheless it is a *practical* disadvantage to be nonpartisan in this debate. It makes one seem remote. Today fanatics get an eager hearing — from exactly the same kind of fanatic. Nothing else will *send* anybody. We listen to ideas as we listen to jazz; we want them to transport us. This is the way things are. People do not even try to be "fair" any more. It seems too professorial. This, not World War I, produced the Lost Generation. This, not World War II, produced the Mislaid Generation. This, not the stuffiness of squares, produces beatniks. To be "beat" is a specialization too, a quest for a personal style so far underwater that any reminder of a community of fellow beings is regarded as an amphibious insult. We secede from society, but we begin by seceding from ourselves.

The effect of this double alienation upon our arts and sciences has received as much critical comment as any other phenomenon of our times. Generally our intellectuals — for example, our obscure poets and our obscure physicists — are attacked as arid and abstract. Actually, however, when they are examined closely they prove to be intensely emotional beings who have crammed lifetimes of feeling into an algebraic poem or a technical book review intelligible to only a few other professionals. Since no steady flow of expression is permitted them by the tight rules of the game they play, they usually have to cede the right to be heard above the crowd to loud-mouthed popularizers who merely translate their ideas into platitudes or megatons. Their ideas are nuggets of feeling that need to be alloyed with baser metals for mass consumption. So our true poets are driven into conversation with one another — in symbols almost as rarely understood as those of the physicists — and run the risk of coterie dry rot unless they can find a way to break their double alienation, from self and society.

Whether Jung's ideas can help them or the scientists remains to be seen. His archetypes are addressed directly to this problem, as a step toward freeing the mind from its immediate surroundings and enabling it to reroot itself in universal history. His typology, with its intricate crisscross of the functions of thought, feeling, intuition, sensation with extroversion and introversion, is also a guide for finding everyman's place in nature. His picture of the feminine portion of man, the *anima,* and the masculine portion of woman, the *animus,* together with his *persona,* or the mask presented to society, and his detailed account of the process of individuation — all of these are so plainly the product of one man's struggle for meaning, with his patients providing the details, that a similarly troubled reader cannot help but follow him with warm sympathy and admiration. "Do not think carnally," he is saying, "or you will be flesh, but think symbolically, and then you will be spirit." If you look clearly at the many determinisms that surround you, you need no longer be at their mercy. You also need not be blindly partisan.

Women will find in Jung an attention to their problems that Adler merely suggests — not their social problems, however, but their personal ones. Much of Jung is addressed to intellectual women who must absorb as harmoniously as possible a disagreeably mannish *animus* if they are to attain their full, complex stature as human beings. Such "priestesses" are subject to much satire from those who would in effect restrict them to the Hitlerian three

K's, but this kind of envious vulgarity means nothing to Jung. He is also not greatly interested in the problems of children, or in the conventional "homemaker"; but unusual women and the fine points of marriage get more attention from him than from any other psychologist. As might be expected from such a curious man, he is also interested in random phenomena that cannot be explained satisfactorily by scientific causality, by possible toxic factors in schizophrenia, by the symbolism of the mass, by the possible relationship of horoscopes to failure in marriage, by the psychic effect of departed redskins on the behavior of present-day American whites. But that is a very small list of his investigations, the broad sweep of which may not have been equaled since the Renaissance.

Possibly the most challenging contribution of Jung is his adaptation of the Polynesian word *mana* (extraphysical power or extraordinary effectiveness) in what he calls "the mana-personality." A few human beings become mana-personalities, he says, through their capacity to control internal forces that formerly may have made their behavior unpredictable but now qualify them to serve as leaders. Such people have descended successfully into their own lower depths, made the "night sea journey" required of the hero, and now they are our best guides. They *know*, they have been there. Nothing human is alien to them. Their humanity is now working *for* them.

Mana is closely related to the "autonomy" that David Riesman expects the lonely crowd to develop: "The very conditions that produce other-direction on the part of the majority today, who are heteronomous — that is, guided by voices other than their own — may also produce a 'saving remnant' who are increasingly autonomous, and who find their strength in the face of their minority position in the modern world of power." But it is not nearly as easy or as vague as that, Jung says. We must acquire an intimate understanding of internal forces that are remarkably similar in everyone. As similar, in fact as the bodily processes of seeing or digestion or breathing. We must wrest power from these internal forces and confer it, not upon a self-inflated ego, but upon our portion of the impersonal. Does it seem simple? It is the most difficult achievement of all.

A Young Psychiatrist Looks at His Profession

ROBERT COLES, M.D.

————•••————

RECENTLY, in the emergency ward of the Children's Hospital in Boston, an eight-year-old girl walked in and asked to talk to a psychiatrist about her "worries." I was called to the ward, and when we ended our conversation I was awake with sorrow and hope for this young girl, but also astonished at her coming. As a child psychiatrist, I was certainly accustomed to the troubled mother who brings her child to a hospital for any one of a wide variety of emotional problems. It was the child's initiative in coming which surprised me. I recalled a story my wife had told me. She was teaching a ninth-grade English class, and they were starting to read the Sophoclean tragedy of *Oedipus*. A worldly thirteen-year-old asked the first question: "What is an Oedipus complex?" Somehow, in our time, psychiatrists have become the heirs of those who hear the worried and see the curious. I wondered, then, what other children in other times did with their troubles and how they talked of the Greeks. I wondered, too, about my own profession, its position and its problems, and about the answers we might have for ourselves as psychiatrists.

We appear in cartoons, on television serials, and in the movies. We are "applied" by Madison Avenue, and we "influence" writers. Acting techniques, even schools of painting, are supposed to be derived from our insights, and Freud has become what Auden calls "a whole climate of opinion." Since children respond so fully to what is most at hand in the adult world, there should have been no reason for my surprise in that emergency ward. But this quick acceptance of us by children and adults alike is ironic, tells us something about this world, and is dangerous.

The irony is that we no longer resemble the small band of outcasts upon whom epithets were hurled for years. One forgets today just how rebellious Freud and his contemporaries were. They studied archaeology and mythology, were versed in the ancient languages, wrote well, and were a bit fiery, a bit eccentric, a bit troublesome, even for one another. Opinionated, determined, oblivious of easy welcome, they were fighters for their beliefs, and their ideas fought much of what the world then thought.

This is a different world. People today are frightened by the memory of concentration camps, by the possibility of atomic war, by the breakdown of old empires and old ways of living and believing. Each person shares the hopes and terrors peculiar to this age, not an age of reason or of enlightenment but an age of fear and trembling. Every year brings problems undreamed of only a decade ago in New York or Vienna. Cultures change radically, values are different, even diseases change. For instance, cases of hysteria, so beautifully described by Freud, are rarely found today. A kind of innocence is lost; people now are less suggestible, less naïve, more devious. They look for help from many sources, and chief among them, psychiatrists. Erich Fromm, in honor of Paul Tillich's seventy-fifth birthday, remarked: "Modern man is lonely, frightened, and hardly capable of love. He wants to be close to his neighbor, and yet he is too unrelated and distant to be able to be close. . . . In search for closeness he craves knowledge; and in search for knowledge he finds psychology. Psychology becomes a substitute for love, for intimacy. . . ."

Now Freud and his knights are dead. Their long fight has won acclaim and increasing protection from a once reluctant society, and perhaps we should expect this ebb tide. Our very acclaim makes us more rigid and querulous. We are rent by rivalries, and early angers or stubborn idiosyncrasies have hardened into a variety of schools with conflicting ideas. We use proper names of early psychiatrists — Jung, Rank, Horney — to describe the slightest differences of emphasis or theory. The public is interested, but understandably confused. If it is any comfort to the public, so are psychiatrists, at times. Most of us can recall our moments of arrogance, only thinly disguised by words which daily become more like shibboleths, sound hollow, and are almost cant.

Ideas need the backing of institutions and firm social approval if they are to result in practical application. Yet I see pharisaic temples being built everywhere in psychiatry; pick up our journals and you will see meetings listed almost every week of the year and pages filled with the abstracts of papers presented at them. These demand precious time in attendance and reading, and such time is squandered all too readily these days. Who of us, even scanting sleep, can keep up with this monthly tidal wave of minute or repetitive studies? And who among us doesn't smile or shrug as he skims the pages, and suddenly leap with hunger at the lonely monograph that really says something? As psychiatrists we need to be in touch not only with our patients but with the entire range of human activity. We need time to see a play or read a poem, yet daily we sit tied to our chairs, listening and talking for hours on end. While this is surely a problem for all professions, it is particularly deadening for one which deals so intimately with people and which requires that its members themselves be alive and alert.

It seems to me that psychiatric institutions and societies too soon become bureaucracies, emphasizing form, detail, and compliance. They also breed the idea that legislation or grants of money for expansion of laboratories and buildings will provide answers where true knowledge is lacking. Whereas we desperately need more money for facilities and training for treatment programs, there can be a vicious circle of more dollars for more specialized projects producing more articles about less and less, and it may be that some projects are contrived to attract money and expand institutions rather than to form any spontaneous intellectual drive. We argue longer and harder about incidentals, such as whether our patients should sit up or lie down; whether we should accept or reject their gifts or answer their letters; how our offices should be decorated; or how we should talk to patients when they arrive or leave. We debate for hours about the difference between psychoanalysis and psychotherapy; about the advantages of seeing a person twice a week or three times a week; about whether we should give medications to people, and if so, in what way. For the plain fact is that as we draw near the bureaucratic and institutionalized, we draw near quibbling. Maybe it is too late, and much of this cannot be stopped. But it may be pleasantly nostalgic, if not instructive, to recall Darwin sailing on the *Beagle*, or Freud writing spirited letters of discovery to a close friend, or Sir Alexander Fleming stumbling upon a mold of penicillin in his laboratory — all in so simple and creative a fashion, and all with so little red tape and money.

If some of psychiatry's problems come from its position in the kind of society we have, other troubles are rooted in the very nature of our job. We labor with people who have troubled thoughts and feelings, who go awry in bed or in the office or with friends. Though we talk a great deal about our scientific interests, man's thoughts and feelings cannot be as easily understood or manipulated as atoms. The brain is where we think and receive impressions of the world, and it is in some ultimate sense an aggregate of atoms and molecules. In time we will know more about how to control and transform all cellular life, and at some point the cells of the brain will be known in all their intricate functions. What we now call ego or unconscious will be understood in terms of cellular action or biochemical and biophysical activity. The logic of the nature of all matter predicts that someday we will be able to arrange and rearrange ideas and feelings. Among the greatest mysteries before us are the unmarked pathways running from the peripheral nervous system to the thinking areas in the brain. The future is even now heralded by machines which think and by drugs which stimulate emotional states or affect specific moods, like depressions. Until these roads are thoroughly surveyed and the brain is completely understood, psychiatry will be as pragmatic or empirical as medicine.

Social scientists have taught us a great deal about how men think and how they get along with one another and develop from infancy to full age. We have learned ways of reaching people with certain problems and can offer much help to some of them. Often we can understand illnesses that we cannot so readily treat. With medicines, we can soften the lacerations of nervousness and fear, producing no solutions, but affording some peace and allowing the mind to seek further aid. Some hospitals now offer carefully planned communities where new friendships can arise, refuges where the unhappy receive individual medical and psychiatric attention. Clinics, though harried by the inadequate size of their staffs and by increasing requests, offer daily help for a variety of mental illnesses. Children come to centers devoted to the study and treatment of early emotional difficulties. If the etiologies are still elusive, the results of treatment are often considerable. Failures are glaring, but the thousands of desperate people who are helped are sometimes overlooked because of their very recovery. Indeed, it is possible that our present problems may give way to worse ones as we get to know more. The enormous difficulties of finding out about the neurophysiology of emotional life may ultimately yield to the Orwellian dilemma of a society in which physicists of the mind can change thoughts and control feelings at their will.

However, right now I think our most pressing concern is less the matter of our work than the manner of ourselves. For the individual psychiatrist, the institutional rigidities affect his thoughts and attitudes, taint his words and feelings, and thereby his ability to treat patients. We become victims of what we most dread; our sensibilities die, and we no longer care or notice. We dread death of the heart — any heart under any moon. Yet I see organization men in psychiatry, with all the problems of death-like conformity. Independent thinking by the adventurous has declined; psychiatric training has become more formal, more preoccupied with certificates and diplomas, more hierarchical. Some of the finest people in early dynamic psychiatry were artists, like Erik Erikson, school-teachers, like August Eichhorn, or those, like Anna Freud, who had no formal training or occupation but motivations as personal as those of a brilliant and loyal daughter. Today we are obsessed with accreditation, recognition, levels of training, with status as scientists. These are the preoccupations of young psychiatrists. There are more lectures, more supervision, more examinations for specialty status, and thus the profession soon attracts people who take to these practices. Once there were the curious and bold; now there are the carefully well-adjusted and certified.

When the heart dies, we slip into wordy and doctrinaire caricatures of life. Our journals, our habits of talk become cluttered with jargon or the trivial. There are negative cathects, libido quanta, "pre-symbiotic, normal-autistic phases of mother-infant unity," and "a hierarchically stratified, firmly cathected organization of self-representations." Such dross is excused as a short cut to understanding a complicated message by those versed in the trade; its practitioners call on the authority of symbolic communication in the sciences. But the real test is whether we best understand by this strange proliferation of language the worries, fears, or loves in individual people. As the words grow longer and the concepts more intricate and tedious, human sorrows and temptations disappear, loves move away, envies and jealousies, revenge and terror dissolve. Gone are strong, sensible words with good meaning and the flavor of the real. Freud called Dostoevsky the greatest psychologist of all time, and long ago Euripedes described in *Medea* the hurt of the mentally ill. Perhaps we cannot expect to describe our patients with the touching accuracy and poetry used for Lady Macbeth or Hamlet or King Lear, but surely there are sparks to be kindled, cries to be heard, from people who are individuals.

If we become cold, and our language frosty, then our estrangement is complete. Living in an unreliable world, often lonely, and for this reason attracted to psychiatry as a job with human contacts, we embrace icy reasoning and abstractions, a desperate shadow of the real friendships which we once desired. Estrangement may, indeed, thread through the entire fabric of our professional lives in America. Cartoons show us pre-empted by the wealthy. The New Haven community study by A. B. Hollingshead and F. C. Redlich, *Social Class and Mental Illness*, shows how few people are reached by psychiatrists, how much a part of the class and caste system in America we are. Separated from us are all the troubled people in villages and farms from Winesburg to Yoknapatawpha. Away from us are the wretched drunks and the youthful gangs in the wilderness of our cities. Removed from us are most of the poor, the criminal, the drug addicts. Though there are some low-cost clinics, their waiting lists are long, and we are all too easily and too often available to the select few of certain streets and certain neighborhoods.

Whereas in Europe the theologian or artist shares intimately with psychiatrists, we stand apart from them, afraid to recognize our common heritage. European psychiatry mingles with philosophers; produces Karl Jaspers, a psychiatrist who is a theologian, or Jean-Paul Sartre, a novelist and philosopher who writes freely and profoundly about psychiatry. After four years of psychiatric training in a not uncultured city, I begin to wonder whether young psychiatrists in America are becoming isolated by an arbitrary definition of what is, in fact, our work. Our work is the human condition, and we might do well to talk with Reinhold Niebuhr about the "nature and destiny of man," or with J. D. Salinger about our Holden Caulfields. Perhaps we are too frightened and too insecure to recognize our very brothers. This is a symptom of the estranged.

In some way our hearts must live. If we truly live, we will talk clearly and avoid the solitary trek. In some way we must manage to blend poetic insight with a craft and unite intimately the rational and the intuitive, the aloof stance of the scholar with the passion and affection of the friend who cares and is moved. It seems to me that this is the oldest summons in the history of Western civilization. We can answer this request only with some capacity for risk, dare, and whim. Thwarting us at every turn of life is the ageless fear of uncertainty; it is hard to risk the unknown. If we see a patient who puzzles us, we can avoid the mystery and challenge of the unique through readily available diagnostic categories. There is no end to classifications and terminologies, but the real end for us may be the soul of man, lost in these words: "Name it and it's so, or call it and it's real." This is the language of children faced with a confusion of the real and unreal, and it is ironic, if human, to see so much of this same habit still among psychiatrists.

Perhaps, if we dared to be free, more would be revealed than we care to admit. I sometimes wonder why we do not have a journal in our profession which publishes anonymous contributions. We might then hear and feel more of the real give-and-take in all those closed offices, get a fuller flavor of the encounter between the two people, patient and psychiatrist, who are in and of themselves what we call psychotherapy. The answer to the skeptic who questions the worth of psychotherapy is neither the withdrawn posture of the adherent of a closed system who dismisses all inquiry as suspect nor an eruption of pseudoscientific verbal pyrotechnics. Problems will not be solved by professional arrogance or more guilds and rituals. For it is more by being than by doing that the meaningful and deeply felt communion between us and our patients will emerge. This demands as much honesty and freedom from us as it does from our patients, and as much trust on our part as we would someday hope to receive from them.

If the patient brings problems that may be understood as similar to those in many others, that may be conceptualized and abstracted, he is still in the midst of a life which is in some ways different from all others. We bring only ourselves; and so each meeting in our long working day is different, and our methods of treatment will differ in many subtle ways from those of all our colleagues. When so much of the world faces the anthill of totalitarian living, it is important for us to affirm proudly the preciously individual in each human being and in ourselves as doctors. When we see patients, the knowledge and wisdom of many intellectual ancestors are in our brains, and hopefully, some life and affection in our hearts. The heart must carry the reasoning across those inches or feet of office room. The psychiatrist, too, has his life and loves, his sorrows and angers. We know that we receive from our patients much of the irrational, misplaced, distorted thoughts and feelings once directed at parents, teachers, brothers, and sisters. We also know that our patients attempt to elicit from us many of the attitudes and responses of these earlier figures. But we must strive for some neutrality, particularly in the beginning of treatment, so that our patients may be offered, through us and their already charged feelings toward us, some idea of past passions presently lived. Yet so often this neutrality becomes our signal for complete anonymity. We try to hide behind our couches, hide ourselves from our patients. In so doing we prolong the very isolation often responsible for our patients' troubles, and if we persist, they will derive from the experience many interpretations but little warmth and trust.

I think that our own lives and problems are part of the therapeutic process. Our feelings, our own disorders and early sorrows are for us in some fashion what the surgeon's skilled hands are for his work. His hands are the trained instruments of knowledge, lectures, traditions. Yet they are, even in surgery, responsive to the artistry, the creative and sensitive intuition of the surgeon as a man. The psychiatrist's hands are himself, his life. We are educated and prepared, able to see and interpret. But we see, talk, and listen through our minds, our memories, our persons. It is through our emotions that the hands of our healing flex and function, reach out, and finally touch.

We cannot solve many problems, and there are the

world and the stars to dwarf us and give us some humor about ourselves. But we can hope that, with some of the feeling of what Martin Buber calls "I-Thou" quietly and lovingly nurtured in some of our patients, there may be more friendliness about us. This would be no small happening, and it is for this that we must work. Alert against dryness and the stale, smiling with others and occasionally at ourselves, we can read and study, but maybe wince, shout, cry, and love, too. Really, there is much less to say than to affirm by living. I would hope that we would dare to accept ourselves fully and offer ourselves freely to a quizzical and apprehensive time and to uneasy and restless people.

The New Drugs

MORTIMER OSTOW, M.D.

————•—•————

TEN years ago, at the age of twenty-two, Mrs. X gave birth to her second baby. Within a week after delivery, she complained that things appeared strange and distant to her. She could not believe that the child was hers. Soon she was convinced that the infant was in some danger, yet she could not bring herself to care for it. A day or so later, she would not move, talk, eat, or care for herself, and she resisted every effort to help her. This was the onset of the first of three attacks of catatonic schizophrenia.

Her husband sought the best professional help available and obtained the assistance of a senior psychiatrist, who promptly hospitalized Mrs. X and instituted a series of twenty electric shock treatments. This procedure induces brief unconsciousness and a convulsion in the patient by the administration of a surge of electricity across the temples. At the rate of three treatments weekly, the series lasted seven weeks, throughout which Mrs. X failed to show the slightest response. She remained in the hospital, and for the next six months underwent a course of insulin coma treatments followed by psychotherapy. Like electric shock, insulin coma also renders the patient unconscious, for an hour or longer; a convulsion may or may not occur. Since Mrs. X continued to be mute during most of this period, I cannot imagine that the psychotherapy consisted of much more than an attempt to establish contact with her and encourage her. Eight months after the onset of her illness, she recovered. Whether the insulin comas or the psychotherapy, or perhaps the combination, effected this remission, who can say? Since then, insulin treatment has lost favor among many psychiatrists; and psychotherapy with mute psychotics, while occasionally effective, is not a patent or reliable therapeutic instrument.

Mrs. X was discharged from the hospital to her home and eagerly resumed her normal activities and obligations. She functioned well, and to all appearances was happy with her husband and children. But five years later, traveling in Europe with her husband, she suddenly displayed the old remote stare, and escaping for a moment from his presence, she swallowed a large amount of the sedative medication her doctor had prescribed for insomnia. Fortunately, this attempt at suicide was ineffective, and the French psychiatrist who was called to treat her administered in daily doses a newly introduced antipsychotic drug, Largactil. In a matter of but a few weeks she recovered completely, and remained well, even after the drug was withdrawn. Apparently the new chemical agent had accomplished, inconspicuously and gently, the same remission of illness that had previously required eight months and many physically jarring procedures. What was the wonder-worker, Largactil?

Largactil is the trade name under which the drug chlorpromazine is marketed in some European countries. Here in the United States it is called Thorazine. It was the first of what has now grown to be a numerous family of antipsychotic drugs, based upon variations of the phenothiazine nucleus. These differ widely in potency, in toxicity, and in their propensity to cause disturbing side effects. But all share the capacity for alleviating psychotic behavior in mania, paranoia, and certain forms of schizophrenia. (It is interesting to note that after more than five years of experience, during which millions of doses have been given, there are still no clear or reliable criteria by which to distinguish between those schizophrenics likely to benefit from Thorazine and those who will not.) In addition to the phenothiazine group, there are two other drugs which exert a similar antipsychotic effect: reserpine, extracted from the plant *Rauwolfia serpentina* and the very first of the antipsychotic pharmaceuticals to be employed clinically; and tetrabenazine. Despite chemical dissimilarities, all three drugs have a common therapeutic effect and common side effects. Together they constitute the widely known family of "tranquilizers."

How do these chemical substances alleviate psychosis? The question readily resolves into two. First, how do these drugs affect the physical organism; and second, how do they affect the psyche, that is, the mental life? We can only guess at answers to both questions. With respect to their organic action, we find, however, a tendency, shared by all three, to produce specific motor effects incidental to their antipsychotic action. Significantly, these same motor disturbances are the symptoms of diseases affecting structures in the brain known as the basal ganglia. The basal ganglia are prominent throughout the vertebrate series and are probably concerned with the regulation of spontaneous activity. Is it not reasonable, then, to infer that the tranquilizers achieve their effect by influencing the function of the basal ganglia?

When we next inquire how the tranquilizers affect the psychic life, we have even less evidence to guide us. We may note that in both animal and man tranquilizers tend to diminish the amount of spontaneous activity and generally to reduce vital functions, including vigor of circulation and respiration, and also body temperature. Employed clinically, the tranquilizers are most likely to be effective in diseases characterized by overactivity, where they reduce the abnormal intensity of striving. Finally, if given in excessive amounts, tranquilizers have been found to produce states of profound mental and physical inertia.

Translating these facts into psychological theory, one may guess that the drugs affect an entity which Freud termed "instinctual energy." Freud hypothesized a certain impetus, a potential for striving, which man's biological nature imposes upon his mind. From this instinctual push, man develops wishes and appetites. Freud observed that it was important to differentiate between two groups of instincts, and therefore between two sources of instinctual energy. There are, first, those instincts which impel an individual to enter into constructive and productive activities, with others. These include social activities, parent-child relationships, courtship and marriage, and even protection, cultivation, and advancement of oneself. These constructive, or "life," instincts are represented in consciousness by the emotion of love, and hence are termed the "erotic instincts"; their energy is known as "libido." The second group of instincts is concerned with death and destruction. If it is true that the tranquilizers reduce the intensity of instinctual energy, it must be primarily, perhaps exclusively, the energy of the erotic instincts that they affect. We have found that when these drugs have been given in amounts sufficient to retard erotic activities or their derivatives, the individual displays anger, fury, and even strong murderous or suicidal tendencies.

We may now ask, how is it that reduction of instinctual impetus can exert a therapeutic effect upon mental illness? Freud provided the answer half a century ago. Mental illness occurs, he said, when instinctual energies accumulate to an intensity too great to be contained by the ego. Freud went even further and predicted that chemical substances would ultimately be found capable of affecting the distribution of energies within the mental apparatus. We would then have a tool for alleviating illnesses so severe as to resist psychoanalysis. In the absence of experimental data, I must emphasize that any attempt to explain the action of the drugs is clearly speculative. While these hypotheses seem the most plausible to me, no one theory has yet found general acceptance among psychiatrists.

To return to Mrs. X: her second recovery was sustained for approximately three years. Becoming aware, then, of inexplicably mounting discontent and apprehension, she turned for treatment to a competent and conscientious psychoanalyst. Dr. Y's psychotherapy was essentially supportive and cautiously avoided any profound psychic exploration aimed at uncovering hidden motivation. He followed accepted practice, which states that in treating an individual who has previously suffered psychosis, any serious attempt to weaken the existing defensive structure invites a breakdown of ego control, with a consequent relapse into psychosis. Unfortunately, the more conservative treatment does not guarantee against relapse either.

One day last June, Mrs. X confided to a friend suspicions that strange men were looking at her and following her in the streets. Within a few hours she had lost contact with reality for the third time and was stopped just as she was about to cut her throat with a kitchen knife. Once again she was hospitalized and subjected to an intensive program of electric shock treatment. Over a period of six weeks, more than sixty convulsions were induced in a desperate effort to dislodge the catatonia. The only persistent effect of the therapy was a painful memory gap. Even today, a year later, long periods of her life and names and identities of many acquaintances remain lost to her. On three occasions she emerged from the schizophrenic attack and seemed well, but the recovery was short-lived and complete relapse occurred within two or three days. You will wonder why she was not given chlorpromazine, which had helped her so readily before. Her doctors did prescribe the drug, but she failed to respond and, in fact, seemed to deteriorate further. Though disappointed, they were not altogether surprised, for experience had taught that not all schizophrenics improve with phenothiazine medication.

What else could be done for her? Following the development of the phenothiazines, it had been observed that an entirely different group of pharmaceutical substances, the psychic energizers, also have a salutary effect upon some schizophrenics. The therapeutic value of these drugs was originally appreciated for the treatment of melancholia. This is a frequent pathological condition characterized by a sense of inner misery, retardation of thought and action, inertia, withdrawal from human company, and a tendency to avoid not only responsibilities and obligations but all pleasurable activities as well. In extreme cases, suicide occurs. Freud suggested that in melancholia the ego is "impoverished," that is, depleted of the psychic energy it requires for normal function. It is consistent with this guess of Freud's that, if administered in excessive doses, the tranquilizers may cause melancholia. The tranquilizers, I believe, reduce the ego's libido content. Psychic energizers, on the other hand, not only relieve melancholia but, in general, reverse the changes that are brought about by tranquilizing medication. For example, a patient who has recovered from mania or schizophrenia with tranquilizing medication will suffer a relapse if then treated with an energizer. The term "psychic energizers" has been applied to this second group of drugs precisely because its members oppose the libido-reducing effects of the tranquilizers and because the conditions they alleviate are uniformly characterized by loss of libido.

The mode of action of the energizers is as mysterious as that of the tranquilizers. Some of the energizers resemble the phenothiazines in chemical structure and occasionally produce similar side effects. It is therefore presumed that they too influence basal ganglia function, but in a direction opposite to the influence of the tranquilizers. Other energizers, quite different chemically, seem to achieve their therapeutic effect by inactivating an enzyme which normally catalyzes one step in the process of protein metabolism. As a result, the concentration in body fluids of certain nitrogenous substances known as amines is increased; it is presumed that this brings about behavioral changes which are best described as the effects of an increase in libido. These are chemical theories which have gained some currency but are far from universally accepted.

When energizers were first employed in the treatment of melancholia, it was found that often, as the melancholia resolved, another illness of neurotic or psychotic proportions was precipitated. From the point of view of clinical therapy, this outcome is considered a side effect or complication of the pharmaceutic treatment. But so drastic a behavioral consequence must also have psychological significance; it must reveal something about the nature of mental illness. One thing is already clear. Various pathological conditions are characterized by an excess of libidinal energy in the ego, while others are characterized by a deficit. We can relieve the former by administering tranquilizers, the latter by administering energizers. It was, however, Freud's original supposition that all mental illness is the consequence of an excessive accumulation of libido within the ego. How, then, can we relate to Freud's theory the fact that there are illnesses — for example, melancholia — in which many of the symptoms are determined by a libido deficiency?

I have speculated that a depletion of the ego occurs normally as a corrective maneuver, whenever the libido content of the ego arises excessively. When this correction fails to occur spontaneously, the ensuing illness may be treated by artificially inducing depletion through the administration of a tranquilizer. The reverse situation, excessive depletion, may also occur, and its pathogenic consequence, melancholia. We can repair the latter by administering an energizer, but by canceling the corrective effect of the initial spontaneous depletion we run the risk of reinducing the original illness — a vicious cycle.

It follows, then, that many patients may be successfully treated only by a combination of energizer and tranquilizer to prevent excessive swings of libido in either direction. It is interesting that when both types of drugs are given simultaneously, in proper dosage, they do not cancel each other's effect, but one acts to provide a floor and the other a ceiling to confine excursions of ego libido within a normal range. Though theoretically simple and straightforward, the actual process of finding the precise balance of tranquilizer and energizer required by any specific patient is difficult and complicated. At present it is achieved only by a method of successive approximation, and we do not know in what proportion of cases it will be successful.

After weeks of treatment with experimental combinations and proportions of drugs, an optimal set was ascertained for Mrs. X, and her profound schizophrenia was dramatically dissipated. But until this was achieved, her behavior ranged from the extremes of inertia, almost lifelessness, to incredible excitement and destructiveness, each state clearly attributable to almost calculable shifts in libido supply. Today Mrs. X is clearly and undeniably well, and it is a good guess that so long as she continues to take the pills that rescued her from illness, she will remain well. Her recovery may even be sustained after medication is discontinued, at least for a while. But the roots of her illness persist, and they will continue to weaken and distort interpersonal relations, specifically the loving relationship with husband and children.

Drug therapy may reverse the severe fluctuations of ego libido that characterize serious neurotic or psychotic breakdown, and it may prevent dangerously great accumulation and depletion, which serve as triggers. But drug therapy cannot correct disturbances of mental function which prevent satisfactory gratification of instinctual needs. Drug therapy can undo the extreme consequences of these dynamic disturbances, but it cannot extirpate the potential for illness, the roots of the disease, the exaggerated unhappiness and the "quiet desperation" of daily life. Against these, only dynamic psychotherapy — definitely, psychoanalysis — is effective.

Through the recognition of distorted patterns of behavior and failure of the capacity to sustain loving relationships, Mrs. X may be led to face her own inner motivations, to uncover destructive goals derived from childhood, to unmask self-deceptions, and to trace their genesis in the past. In this living and intensive observing and remembering, she will begin to find her way to satisfactions she had previously avoided and simultaneously to lose interest in substitutes, which at best rob life of its richness and pleasure and at worst lead to serious illness and suicide. If the psychoanalysis is successful, it should become possible to withdraw the medication and leave Mrs. X immune to relapse.

It should be clear that all aspects of mental illness cannot be comprehended in terms of drug therapy. The germs of mental illness begin to grow in the individual's childhood, and its specific manifestations are determined by his personal experiences. Under what circumstances the illness will appear is dictated by his current problems. During the course of the illness itself, every symptom is the result of three sets of factors: genetic, that is, the individual's childhood experience; dynamic, his current temptations, frustrations, and inhibitions; and energetic. To be entirely correct, one should probably mention constitutional factors as well, but we cannot yet deal with these independently of the others.

Dramatic as has been the change in prognosis for the individual psychotic patient, an even vaster revolution has taken place throughout the whole of psychiatric practice and theory. The fact that it has occurred in precincts normally isolated from general view — the mental hospital, the psychiatrist's office, the laboratory, and the scientific meeting — has perhaps obscured its full significance. First, and probably foremost, the drugs have brought under some control the constantly increasing population of psychiatric hospitals. Many psychotic patients for whom there was formerly no alternative to protracted institutionalization may now be relieved in the early stages of illness. A good number may be treated at home and spared hospitalization altogether, since the threat of suicide and of destructive behavior may be minimized fairly rapidly. In some instances, even addictions may be terminated, perverse behavior and antisocial impulses tamed.

For those who cannot safely remain in society, the average hospital stay has been sharply reduced. Hospital functions and procedures for the acutely ill are, in turn, undergoing radical revision. No longer preoccupied with custodial care, an institutional staff may now exploit to a far greater degree occupational therapy, recreational activities, and classroom instruction. There is a steady decrease in the frequency of those time-honored horrors of mental hospitalization: disturbed wards, restraining camisoles, and sedative baths. The effort to treat the mentally ill in open, rather than locked, wards has similarly been facilitated by the advent of drug therapy. Reduction in hospitalization time and control of destructive behavior have encouraged the treatment of acute mental illness in centrally located general hospitals rather than in country sanitariums. Further, the high financial cost of mental illness, directly in terms of hospital and professional charges, indirectly in protracted loss of working capacity and income, has been substantially reduced.

That the method is only 50 or 60 or 70 per cent effective, that in many instances it limits the extent of deterioration but does not cure, indicate that we are dealing with therapies rather than with miracles, and with human beings rather than with inert laboratory materials. What has been achieved is important, but we also need to improve our techniques for employing the agents we now possess. Poor understanding of just what we are doing with these substances and how we are doing it is, in my opinion, the chief limit to their effectiveness today.

The development of the newer drugs has profound implications for the practice of psychotherapy and psychoanalysis too. Perhaps the most serious intrinsic limitation of psychotherapy has been its inapplicability to the major psychoses and several other categories of illness. By combining drug treatment with psychotherapy, it is possible to establish and to guarantee the minimal psychic stability required for the effective conduct of psychotherapy. Traditionally inaccessible patients may now be inducted into psychotherapy and maintained within a reasonable working range, protected against relapse. Not only may the active psychotic be relieved of his symptoms and initiated into psychotherapy, but the psychotic in remission, the interval personality, may be treated psychotherapeutically without fear of inducing further breakdown. And the occasional psychosis, the schizophrenia or melancholia which supervenes under analysis or psychotherapy, may now be handled without arresting, even temporarily, the psychotherapy. Thus, the spectrum of disorders amenable to definitive therapy becomes considerably broadened, and direct psychological observation and study of psychosis and the psychotic process become possible. In fact, such close study is inevitable, for the only rational administration of drugs must be in accordance with specific psychological criteria, irrespective of symptomatology.

It would be less than objective to omit mention of the limitations of drug therapy, alone or in combination with psychotherapy. Chief among these is its inapplicability to most patients with neurotic disorders. It does not influence the difficulty in interpersonal relations which results from the pathogenic process but which does not seem to signify disease so obviously as frank symptoms. When the neurosis is treated psychotherapeutically and dynamic changes invoke energetic perturbations, drugs are virtually useless. The spontaneous deviations are so small and the equilibrium so fluid that even a small pharmaceutic push easily causes an inordinate swing from which a second set of symptoms evolves and replaces those symptoms that have been relieved. In many other conditions that are responsive to drugs, management of the drug therapy may be difficult. The proper selection, dosage, combination, and sequence of drugs are often a complex and subtle problem. Toxic and side effects sometimes seriously complicate the treatment, and the period of latency — occasionally five weeks or more — before the appearance of any clinical improvement often constitutes a hazard for the suicidal or seriously disturbed patient. And, finally, there is the omnipresent danger of unwise use. The easy promise of relief may seduce the physician and cause him to lose interest in the psychological aspect of mental illness and to minimize the problems of the interval personality. He may consider it unnecessary to view the patient within the context of family relations and be satisfied to cope with a breakdown when it occurs rather than treat the basic pathology.

But, withal, drug therapy has provided the first new tool of major significance for the treatment and understanding of mental illness in several decades. I would find it difficult to overestimate its role in psychiatric and psychoanalytic practice and theory in the years to come.

The Neurotic's Notebook

MIGNON McLAUGHLIN

———•••———

If you had an unhappy childhood, you will always want to sleep late in the morning.

It must infuriate our children to see us always so much more forbearing with everybody else's.

The two unhappiest years in a woman's life: when she is thirteen, and when her daughter is.

Neurotics love being in debt; it proves that someone trusts them.

When men complain that they don't understand women, they mean they don't want to be bothered trying.

The mark of the neurotic: to imagine that you're the only one who cares deeply about anything.

My right hand knows what my left is doing, but is too fine to do it.

The neurotic longs to touch bottom, so at least he won't have *that* to worry about any more.

Neurotics are always afraid of missing something: a remark, a reward, a reprieve.

The neurotic has perfect vision in one eye, but he cannot remember which.

We hear only half of what is said to us, understand only half of that, believe only half of that, and remember only half of that.

It's axiomatic, in geometry, that a thing is always equal to itself. But any neurotic can tell you better, for he is not.

"Pull yourself together" is seldom said to anyone who can.

Throughout our lives, we see in the mirror the same innocent trusting face we have seen there since childhood.

Don't ask others to forgive in you a sin they're dying to commit themselves.

The neurotic is always leaning on someone who is already leaning on someone else.

The fault no child ever loses is the one he was most punished for.

PART II

Psychiatry and Society

The Century of the Child

PETER B. NEUBAUER, M.D.

T HE scientific study of child development did not begin until the twentieth century, which has been called, among other things, the Century of the Child. If it is to live up to this label, we must make better use of the next forty years than we have of the past sixty. But the revolution in child psychiatry is still relatively young, and I will begin by trying to sketch the somewhat erratic course it has taken so far.

If I dwell on the thought and influence of Freud, it is because I speak as a child psychiatrist; but I do not wish to minimize the contribution which outstanding people in other disciplines have made to our understanding of childhood. Jean Piaget and Robert Sears in the field of psychology, Margaret Mead in anthropology, Konrad Lorenz in ethology, and the Russian Pavlovians are a few of the people that come readily to mind. Freud, however, was the first to attempt to give us a body of scientific knowledge that would lead to a general psychology of man. The anthropologists, applying this knowledge to the study of culture and society, found that child-rearing processes furnished illuminating clues to an understanding of people and their institutions. The pediatricians learned to connect physical growth with emotional development, and the way was paved for Dr. Benjamin Spock to write his bible on the subject of infant care. Whichever way we turn, we detect the seminal influence of Freud's discoveries.

Freud's investigations into the neuroses of adults forced him to reconstruct their early childhoods and provided clinical support for the old belief that "The child is the father of the man." His findings led him to frame not only a psychology of man but also laws of human development, and his contributions have completely changed our image of childhood. Gone is the sentimental view that childhood is an era of innocence and the belief that an innate process of development continuously unfolds along more or less immutable lines. Freud suggested that, from birth on, the child's development proceeds in a succession of well-defined stages, each with its own distinctive psychic organization, and that at each stage environmental factors can foster health and achievement or bring about lasting retardation and pathology.

This realization has placed new and complex responsibilities on parents, teachers, and community services. Many parents are now well aware how much their presence or absence, their words, their actions — indeed, their whole emotional state — affect their children. This is an important gain. Unfortunately, it must be added that Freud's theories have also been widely misunderstood. For one thing, they have been taken to mean that discipline should be suspended, controls eliminated — in sum, that the child should be continuously gratified. Freud, on the contrary, pointed out that denial and conflict were as essential a part of the process of growth as gratification, and he never minimized the child's need for direction.

There are two main reasons why this aspect of Freudian doctrine has been so seriously misinterpreted. In the first place, his early studies of neurosis, made in the bourgeois culture of the late Victorian era, brought to light the damaging effects of authoritarian parental control, moral overrestriction, and stifling prudery; and it was no doubt inevitable that his emancipatory discoveries should have encouraged a concept of child rearing which went overboard on the side of permissiveness.

A second reason for the confusion which has arisen is to be found in the path followed by Freud's own thought. In the early years, he concentrated on those factors in neurosis which stemmed from abnormal repression of the instinctual drives, the forces of the id. It was not until the 1920s that he shifted the main focus of his investigations from the id to the role of the ego — the managerial aspect of man's psychic structure which seeks to align his instinctual drives and moral imperatives with reality. Now, when Freud's doctrine began to be widely propagated in the 1920s, its publicists and popularizers were, at best, familiar only with his early work. They were the spokesmen of a cultural revolt which sought to discredit the moral prohibitions of the past, and they presented an often garbled version of Freud's early findings as a scientific justification of the cult of uninhibited "self-expression." Even today, few laymen are well acquainted with Freud's ego psychology, which emphasizes the organizing and integrating aspects of the ego. These later theories are very important to our understanding of the child. They show that the ego is not self-formative, and they clearly imply that the answer to the crippling restrictiveness of the past is not its diametric opposite, unqualified license.

In fact, Freudian psychology does not, as some people apparently imagine, provide a set of ready-made prescriptions for the rearing of children. It has forced us to take into account not only what the mother or teacher does to a child, but also how it is done; not only whether the mother nurses the baby and spends much time with him, but also whether she is able to give him gratification and support his strivings for mastery. The complexity of the interactions between mother and child cannot be reduced to rigid formulas. Love and understanding cannot be prescribed, and if they are not genuinely manifested, the most enlightened efforts to do what is best for the child may not be effective.

It is certainly encouraging to see how eager are millions of parents today to learn how they can contribute most to the development of their children; the upsurge of interest in this field is nothing less than extraordinary. But a note of caution must be sounded. It is a mistake to look for clear-cut, universal answers on such issues as schedule feeding versus demand feeding, imposed toilet training versus demand training, discipline versus self-regulation. In every case, individual factors are involved, and one needs to know the specific quality of the parent-child relationship before recommendations can safely be made. The newspaper or magazine columnists who impersonally dispense answers to their readers' queries are likely to oversimplify the problems, and their advice could readily be misleading. The whole of Freud's contribution points up the complexity of human nature and the intricacy of the laws which govern the early phases of development. Whoever has understood a single page of Freud knows that he never dealt in facile prescriptions.

It is only in recent years that child psychiatry — the term was first used in 1935 — has become recognized as a specialty in its own right. In the past, children were treated as though they were small adults. Their mental disorders were approached with the same criteria as those clinically applied to adults; it was not realized that the same disorder manifests itself differently in a child than in a grown-up person, because the child's organism is different. Thus, until two decades ago, no one diagnosed schizophrenia in childhood, owing to the fact that the expected symptoms were not encountered. But systematic observation of children from birth on has enlarged our understanding of child development, and one of the consequences of our new knowledge is the discovery of schizophrenia in childhood. Indeed, tremendous progress has been made in helping schizophrenic children, even though the precise cause of the disease remains obscure.

Twenty years ago, very little was known about the nature of mental deficiency; children suffering from a wide variety of ills were lumped together as "mentally defective." Now mental deficiency is in the foreground of investigation and has been broken down into at least fifty categories. We have discovered many of the specific biological disorders which underlie some of these categories, and this is a first step toward devising appropriate treatment. Character disorders and the forerunners of neurotic symptoms can now be detected in the first few years of life. We have understood that they are bound up with specific life situations to which a child is struggling to adjust, and we treat them with encouraging results. There have been studies of normal children who have to make an adjustment to pathology in the family or to a pernicious environment; of children whose own weaknesses, coupled with bad environmental conditions, are leading them into emotional pathology; and of children who are deeply disturbed within a normal environment.

Many research studies are collecting data which will corroborate, modify, or put in question our theories. Most of the studies are based on few cases, but each child is explored as intensively as possible. We hope that these researches will teach us more about the nature of native endowment and thereby help us to understand why various children react so differently to the same environment. Already we have been able to make a beginning toward classifying different patterns of functioning. These delineations of various types of children, based on intensive study of their psychic biographies, should eventually lead to far-reaching changes in child rearing. We will not treat the child according to general principles of what is "good for children," but will pay far greater attention to the differing needs of children with different native endowments.

A good example of the high cost of failure in this sphere is the problem of juvenile delinquency, which underlines the urgency of applying on a larger scale our existing knowledge about the causes of antisocial behavior. We do not, to be sure, know all of the factors involved in such behavior. But it is well established that its main sources are a disrupted home and a bad environment, which combine to prevent normal integration. If we were to tackle individual and social pathology early enough, the incidence of juvenile delinquency could be substantially decreased. Unfortunately, the emergency programs that are currently being applied are not infrequently confused or inappropriate.

One trouble is that the term "juvenile delinquency" fails

to differentiate between the various sources of antisocial behavior. The delinquent may be suffering from a neurotic conflict in which aggression is wildly mobilized against society; he may be a young psychopath who has never developed an adequate sense of right and wrong — in clinical terms, he has a deficient superego. He may be suffering from organic difficulties which make him a slavish follower who simply carries out actions planned and directed by others. He may be an adolescent whose behavior reflects the pathology of his environment rather than any defect in his own psychic structure. Clearly, for each of the cases enumerated, different measures are required. To lump a variety of quite different problems, individual and social, under an oversimplified heading and apply to them the same program is not a particularly promising line of attack.

I said at the outset that we must make better use of the next forty years than we have of the past sixty if the twentieth century is really to be the century of the child. In November, 1959, the United Nations adopted a Declaration of the Rights of the Child, setting forth the rights and freedoms which every child should enjoy. The minimal conditions outlined in the declaration are a far-distant ideal for much of the world's child population. Even in a country as rich and advanced as the United States, two million children live in destitution in homes in which a parent is absent or ill. It is estimated that more than half the children in foster care are emotionally disturbed, and for many of them the only professional help available is a social caseworker. Their disturbances are not temporary, like scarlet fever; they are conditions which will permanently affect the welfare of the child and the nation.

Four fifths of all counties in the United States still have no psychiatric services whatsoever. Fifty per cent of all clinics are concentrated in the Northeastern states, and only 3 per cent of all psychiatric clinical services are located in areas with a population of under twenty-five hundred. Studies of school children in various cities indicate that 7 to 12 per cent of them — that is to say, between two and four million — are in need of psychiatric treatment.

The knowledge we have accumulated points up the importance of organizing resources for the protection and care of the very young child, and here our performance has been especially inadequate. The very young child does not ask for help; it is the responsibility of adults to recognize his need for it. But most parents, when they detect signs of emotional disturbance in a small child, assume — or, at any rate, hope — that he will somehow outgrow it. Thus, nearly all of the children who come to our professional attention are over the age of six, by which time their distress is so acute that parents or teachers can no longer avoid doing something about it. The situation is aggravated by the fact that even among child psychiatrists there are few who have been specially trained to treat the child of preschool age.

Perhaps the greatest lag in the field of mental health is the relative lack of action to implement our conviction that emotional health and pathology are determined in early childhood. More than half of all hospital beds in the United States are occupied by mentally ill patients, yet there exist almost no institutional facilities for the emotionally disturbed preschool child. As long as we neglect the needs of the very young, we will continue to have a large population of adolescents and adults suffering from neurosis or the acuter forms of mental illness.

It seems to me not utopian to suggest that every community of a certain size should have a child health center, which would be equipped to diagnose and treat early disturbances, would assemble data of value to researchers, and would collaborate in various ways with nursery schools, social workers, child guidance services, and psychiatric clinics. We need, also, to set up research centers exclusively concerned with child development, where anthropologists, educators, pediatricians, psychologists, and psychiatrists would have opportunities to join in long-range systematic research.

In psychiatry, as in other fields, the great advances in the application of knowledge have usually come through social change rather than through the immediate pressure of professional people. The French Revolution freed the mentally ill from chains and prisons. The progress recently made in the mental health movement was spurred by the wartime need for total mobilization; of the millions screened, so many were found to be uneducated or emotionally disturbed that the government was forced to concern itself more seriously with the quality of its manpower. Now President Kennedy has established a child health center, which engages in interdisciplinary research, mainly on the problem of mental retardation. This is an encouraging step. One can only hope that it is the beginning of public policies which will carry the thinking of the New Frontier over into the field of child psychiatry.

The Americanization of the Unconscious

JOHN R. SEELEY

———•———

AMERICA is the world's Wonderland. In all the shadings and nuances of the word, she is before all others the world's producer of wonders and is a matter of wonder to the alien, and, *a fortiori,* to herself. Of only one thing can we be sure: that the face she presents to the world — the simple, plain-spoken, direct, homely, straightforward, practical face — is the least of her aspects and serves chiefly to conceal the complexity within complexity that is characteristically hers. Like the latest bikini, the myth of simplicity which she has woven about herself and persuaded others to weave about her calls attention most to what it is ostensibly designed to conceal.

The love affair between America and its image is unlike any other under the moon or sun. Other nations hold before them for relatively lengthy periods rather steady images of their own collective personality, clear-eyed or distorted. Some move from phases of self-glorification to phases of self-denigration: from Rudyard Kipling, say, to the Angry Young Men. Some brood endlessly on the mystery of their being, sinking deeper into a mystery that is always the same. Some romanticize, or, as in Canada, pursue frantically a national identity which eludes perception because it is pursued. But only in America does one turn and turn the corporate image before all the available transforming mirrors of this frame of reference and that. Other peoples glory also in their singularity, but since the singularity of America is its variation, how could America fail to glory precisely in that?

An air of messianic expectation pervades the culture, as one would expect in a society where the conventional belief is in fundamental equality. The log cabin to White House legend masks rather than reveals the much deeper conviction that some much more general and profound savior from something more pervasive than the moment's political problems will at any moment appear and be recognized. The excessive and unadmitted expectation accounts in part for the typically rapid rise and fall of the hero: overrapid rise because the expectation creates the necessity of projecting onto the candidate the preshaped halo; overrapid fall because such distortion of reality cannot be long maintained. (I know the habit is to account for such phenomena in terms of the highly developed communications media, the maneuvers of publicity, the harsh glare of the spotlight. But the media are the means, not the purpose. One does not develop a far-flung net of detection to observe what is not of paramount interest.)

It is true, no doubt, that to a very large extent Americans have made what they call "religion" shallow, but it would be only a slight exaggeration to say that Americans are the most unsecular people on earth. If devotion to an idea, if ardor in its affectionate development, if the rendering of the idea immanent in the body of thought of the time, and if the pervasive embodiment of the idea in behavior are, as I believe, the hallmarks of a "religious" attitude toward it, then ideas are religiously treated in America. It is true that one religion rather readily succeeds another, but this is rather from the devotion to the general religious quest than from disloyalty to the particular religion abandoned. "God by God goes out, discrowned and disanointed, But the soul stands fast that gave them shape and speech."

Lastly, contradictory but coexistent, just as everyone who is anyone becomes a hero, so everything that is anything tends to become an industry. By an "industry" I mean nothing more than some enormous organization in which some input is put in, brought under a rational process, characterized by a maximum of rationality (minute subdivision of labor, immense organization, and exact adaptation of calculated means to ends), and thereby some output is put out. Whether the matter is child raising, or higher education, or entertainment, or the production of a new generation of non-Momistic mothers — or even religion, in the narrower sense — almost inevitably it is so organized and so put into production.

Into a culture so constituted in its general workings was implanted, about 1909, a cultural seedling, the thought and technique of Sigmund Freud. In almost any soil, the seedling was bound to become a mustard tree, with room for all manner of fowl to lodge in. In America it was to transform and be transformed by the society.

The *practice* of psychoanalysis underwent almost no change in the transplantation, except that for reasons which have more to do with politics than culture, it fell almost exclusively into the hands of doctors. (It should be remembered that Freud to his life's end tried to live down his definition and attitude as a physician in favor of a redefinition as a psychologist-philosopher of theory and unquestionably a prophet-priest of practice.) It was the theory, by far the more important part, that was to be modified and made over, and to modify and make over men, theories, and institutions.

Freud's doctrines, as they reached these shores, were by implication stern, if not gloomy. Since his writings fill a good-sized shelf, it would seem idle to attempt to reduce them to a paragraph. The leading ideas that are of interest here concern the instinct theory, the "institutions of the psyche," and the nature of man and society.

Man, as Freud portrayed him, comes to the world panoplied with a full accouterment of instinctual drives. Pleasure (or happiness) lies in the satisfaction and gratification of these instinctual demands, which are in principle insatiable; more particularly, the pandemic demands are for outlets for sexuality and aggression. It is in the very nature of man, in Freud's view, that he cannot live outside society, while at the same time it is in the very nature of society to require renunciation of instinctual gratification, the only source of happiness. Since society cannot survive without taming the instinctual demands, and indeed subverting them to its uses, it achieves its ends, at the expense of individual happiness, by routinely, radically, and inevitably dividing the psyche against itself. This double assault upon the possibility of any sensible degree of happiness — the truncating of the individual's opportunities for gratification, together with the internalization within him of the conflict that "really" lies between him and his fellows — is carried out upon the helpless infant by the unwitting adults.

The first figure in the drama of the child's ontogeny is the id, an institution of the psyche, largely unconscious,

representing in principle unlimited demand for the gratification of sexual and aggressive instincts. The nature of
the environment requires from the child sufficient appreciation of that which is independent of his wishes that he
does not totally stultify his own search for gratification
by the use of inappropriate means. A second institution,
custodian of the "reality principle," is thus differentiated
in the ego. But dominant in the child's significant environment are those who can and do most obviously give
and withhold gratification, mete out reward and punishment; the custodians of the culture, the surrogates for the
society's interests, the parents or their deputies.

In the course of time, the watching, warding, judging,
criticizing, ruling, governing behavior of these virtual jail-
keepers of the instincts is internalized in yet a third institution, differentiated from and set over against the ego,
the superego, again mostly unconscious, but none the less
censorious, vigilant, and punitive. The ego now has an
additional reality to deal with, the conflict between the
excessive demands of the id for gratification and of the
superego for the limiting or extinction of these demands.
A great deal of the limited energy available to the ego is
thus consumed in ceaseless adjudication between one
party, that would empty life of pleasure, and the other,
that would rob it of safety. The child is finally his own
prisoner, jailer, and the mediator between the two. By a
final and exquisitely ironic twist, the very aggression that
is thus cut off from its gratification becomes the very
source of the energy of the superego, so that the psyche
is indeed "the plough-cloven clod/And the ploughshare
drawn thorough." What is to be inferred with regard to
man and society, Freud says in one of the starkest of his
works, *Civilization and Its Discontents*. The burden of

the volume is that, as man seeks to defend himself against disaster-bearing nature and against the disease- and death-bearing body, the very necessities of the defense organization (society and culture) require the attenuation of sources of satisfaction to such a degree that the life thus secured is mostly precarious and, even when stable, scarcely to be endured. He leaves both the survival of civilization and the capacity of men to survive under it as open questions.

The popular myth is that these gloomy doctrines, running into the irrepressible optimism and meliorism of the American people, underwent characteristically American reversals and came out transformed, pupa into butterfly, in the much more palatable dogmas of those who were politely called the revisionists: Horney, Fromm, Sullivan, and others. It is true that a "revision" occurred, a revision perhaps as radical as the one that produced Marxian materialism out of Hegelian idealism; but what made the revision possible and necessary had little to do with American optimism directly. In any case, what is most interesting and most American is not the revision as such but the subsequent "psychoanalyzation" — horrible coinage, but what word will serve? — of American thought, institutions, and life.

In the first place, the words were hardly cool on Freud's lips, the ink hardly dry on his pen, before revisionism — or, as he looked upon it, apostasy — set in, even in Europe. Jung, Adler, Ferenczi, Reich, Reik, Rank and Stekel were the most eminent of Freud's disciples to break away from him. In a sense — though tragically, he did not see it so — revision was a movement that the master himself set off, both by his method and the power of example, and he had as much chance of stopping it as Luther had of limiting Protestantism to his own first great protest. So the fact of revision is not purely American.

Nor is the direction taken by revision so easily to be explained. Horney, Sullivan, and Fromm each developed a connected viewpoint, either implicit or explicit, and in the case of Sullivan, the least known of the three, something that approached a new systematics. More of Freud survives in all three than any one of them is ready to admit; so much, indeed, that one can see a distant ecumenical reunion, perhaps a century off. What binds the major revisionist schools together is a sizable shift from a biological determinism toward a cultural and social determinism, together with a preoccupation with the self as the unit of concern and investigation, the central element in theory, in contradistinction to the preoccupation with the fate of instincts and the squabbles of the psychic trinity. This is not to say, of course, that any of the revisers denies instincts, though all reduce the role played by infantile sexuality and aggression. But what was peripheral in Freud's developed work — ego function, the role of ego ideals, and so forth — becomes central for the three; and what was central for Freud becomes peripheral.

Since society and social relations — "interpersonal relations," as Sullivan significantly calls them — are thought to be more readily amenable to rational improvement than biologically given instincts, there is unquestionably a greater air of optimism in what the revisionists say and an unmistakable foundation for meliorism for those so inclined. Indeed, in Erich Fromm, the message very nearly moves from historical analysis, in *Escape from Freedom*, to a combination of character typology, philosophy, and institutional analysis in *Man for Himself*, to a virtual trumpet call to a quite particular social reform as the means to psychological health in *The Sane Society*.

What made this particular line of revision necessary and possible was the prior existence in America of a fairly well-developed body of fact and theory in the social sciences generally, more particularly in sociology, anthropology, and social psychology. It was the collision with this rival episcopate, already considerably entrenched in American affections, already holding up its crosier over American life, and already holding out the promise of offering America more images of more of its illimitable aspects, that gave the revisionists the impulse, the possibility, and the model for their subsequent development. The existence of this body of specialists, their particular orientations, and the actual and potential public interest in them are, of course, consequences of American affluence, the necessities of self-understanding posed by the melting pot, by rapid social mobility, and by all the characteristics of American culture pointed to at the beginning of this article. But it was the collision of European psychoanalytic theory and case material with American social and social-psychological theory that gave the revision its form and preoccupation and part of its content. From the time of the collision, neither was ever again quite the same. Much social science continued with studied inattention to psychoanalytic theory; some psychoanalytic theory continued in studied disregard of social science; but a great deal of each now took a new turn, fertilized by the other, and out of the fertilization grew a new child that might be labeled either social-psychoanalytic theory or psychoanalytic-social theory.

It is hard to see how, in a social-scientific community sensitized by the work of a long line of social psychologists, reaching from James Mark Baldwin to George Herbert Mead, the central problem of the organization of the self, stated in terms of role taking and role generalization, could be long evaded by any group claiming to understand the genesis of personality. The interest of Charles Horton Cooley in the "primary group" and its relation to the "social self" was contributory to the focus on "interpersonal relations" which Sullivan was so expertly to fill out. The hard-won anthropological and sociological materials were ready to cross-question any general theory of human nature or human development that was too narrowly based on a single society, a single class, or an otherwise biased sample. Each parent needed what the other had: adequate case materials, particularly of sufficient depth and intimacy, were lacking to give body to the rather lofty generalizations of social psychology; adequate formalization of the relation between social process and psychological process had been lacking in most psychoanalytic thought.

The interplay between social science and psychoanalytic theory becomes too complex to follow much further. It results at one point in the anthropologically informed psychological theories of social character of an Abraham Kardiner, the psychoanalytically sensitized anthropology of a Margaret Mead, the revisionist sensitized social character typology of a David Riesman, the exquisitely sensitive playing back and forth between person and society, concrete and particularized, rather than abstract and general, of an Erik Erikson.

In a fashion somehow also typically American, orthodox Freudianism survives and develops. There is intersect antipathy, but, characteristically, there are no wars of religion. Indeed, the true church not only survives and develops, it flourishes, is favored by the hard-core social scientists over the offerings of the revisionists, who are rejected partly on intellectual grounds and partly on the emotional ground that they make things, including the life of the social scientist, too easy. The psychoanalysts come to terms with what David Riesman has called the "dirty secrets" of sociology — social class, ethnicity, and the like; the sociologists come to terms with the corresponding dirty secrets of the analysts — sex and aggression. The preoccupation of each with the supposed preoccupation of the other can be explained sociologically or psychoanalytically and appears equally interesting either way.

Much more dramatic than any of this analysis of analysis and its fate among the professionals is the story of its destiny and development into something immanent in American life, interfused with all thought and activity, making over the society in as radical — and as shallow — a way as the official religions had done earlier: Christianity and liberal, capitalist democracy.

Perhaps this is the point at which to set up some contrasts with Europe, which I toured one summer with one question in mind: How far had the views and preoccupation of mental health spread, ramified, infused the views of educators, city planners, makers of social policy generally, parents, writers, politicians, administrators, executives, and so on — in short, nonpsychiatrists?

In the first place, they had access to, had read, and were highly interested in our social science and psychoanalytic literature, American and — what there is of it — Canadian. They regarded it predominantly in a detached way: an interesting expression, symbolically, of America, no doubt, and a good enough account of American life, but neither directly applicable to them nor providing a model which they might apply to their own self-study. (Actually, excellent similar studies had been made of European life by Europeans, but they were less widely known or appreciated.)

We found excellent mental health enterprises — indeed, some so excellent that the best in America suffer, I think, by comparison — but little or no tendency to generalize, either by reproducing rapidly copies of the dramatically successful enterprises or by "drawing out their principles" and seeking to apply them over a wide range of life, let alone re-examining general social objectives in the light of them. We found remarkably good research, but the people who knew or cared about it were largely the professionals, and then either, as in England, in a task-oriented sense or, as in Germany, in a dominantly philosophical one. It is as though the movements of thought which in America are almost instantaneously communicated to every cell of the body — a sort of intellectual-emotional metastasis — were there localized and only allowed to exert a general influence gradually, if at all. The remark of a very literate, sophisticated old schoolteacher may be allowed to stand as typical: Yes, she knew a good deal about Freud; no, it had little to do with the bringing up of children. We found the same sharp split in France between problems of therapy and problems of development. Our teacher and her contemporaries had even once taken a course on the *Geisteskrankenheiten,* but she spoke of it with the same reminiscent delight and the same air of separation from the everyday concerns of life as if she had been speaking of a course in Egyptian hieroglyphics. In fact it had for her something of just that travelogue quality: interesting, quaint, but happily remote, and someone else's worry.

More typical of America would be to take one institution, the school, faintly adumbrated in *Crestwood Heights,* but to be found in pure form in numberless suburbs.

In the pure form, not only means and methods but goals and criteria of performance have been made over in terms of available psychoanalytic understandings. Just as religion has become a way to peace of mind, thereby emptying it of specifically religious content, so education has become the way to strength of soul, to positive mental health, to maturity. It is not that teachers are preoccupied by pathology; they are too healthy for that, though their rather general viewing of children as problems — parallelled by parent perceptions in the same terms — begins to border on that danger. It is rather that everything is seen, understood, and acted upon, as far as reality permits, in terms of the depth drama actually or possibly underlying any act. Little behavior is taken at face value; almost without consciousness of alternate possibilities of perception, very nearly everything is *interpreted.* The role of the teacher as a parent surrogate is understood and accepted. It is expected that hostility will be displaced upon her, that drawings, essays, polite exchanges have covert meanings much different from their overt content — and much more real and much more interesting. The libidinal give-and-take that accompanies all communication (or motivates it?) is noted, although less easily accepted. If Johnny throws a spitball at Mary, nothing so ordinary as mischief is afoot. The possibilities have to be — are joyously — entertained that Johnny is working off aggression, compensating for deeply felt inferiority, asserting his masculinity in ways appropriate to his developmental stage, testing for limits, or, in a characteristic upside-down way, saying to Mary in a circuitous and hence safe way, "I love you."

And so, not only for students, but for the interrelations of staff and of all to authority. The mental health of the staff as a prerequisite for the mental health of the pupils is a matter of concern — not, of course, in the bare sense that teachers should not be mentally sick, but that they also should be positively well, continuously growing, always developing and maturing, and manifestly happy, continuously emotionally rewarded in so doing. I will not go on. The rest spells itself out. Except, perhaps, that I should note that in such schools the parents — or, at least, the mothers — must be continuously caught up in the enterprise to a point of unexampled intimacy and in a role partly of lay assistants in the child's upbringing and partly of apprentices or pupils.

What is true for the school is true for the church, for industry — on the white-collar side, at least — for the family, and even, to a sensible degree, for the peer-group institutions among the youngsters themselves. The explicit awareness of high school kids — and those in the elementary school, down to kindergarten — of the depth-psychological world they now inhabit is exquisite, and many of them know their gamesmanship better than the adults.

This development in America, and it has still to run the major part of its course, makes for a change in the very nature of the society, comparable in the magnitude of its effect to the original American Revolution. But that was a revolution of mere *externa*: this is of *interna, ultima, privatissima*. We are confronted by the possibility — perhaps, now, the inescapable necessity — of a highly self-

conscious society of highly self-conscious individuals, a
society that must sustain, cope with, or use all the new
possibilities of vertical complexity in addition to the pre-
existing ones of horizontal complexity. We have added a
dimension, and there is no more radical act. We are in the
process of producing, if we have not already produced, a
distinctly American unconscious.

Such a society has the possibility of approximating a
therapeutic community, or, rather, a community favor-
able to the emergence of a humanity more humane than
any we have ever known. It has also the possibility of
becoming a manipulative society in which the minor,
clumsy attempts depicted by Vance Packard in *The Hidden Persuaders* are perfected to the point where resistance
is virtually meaningless; a society in which, moreover, the
threats of manipulation from without are countered but
fatally compounded by self-manipulation, which is also in
the current American stream. The dice are heavily loaded
in favor of the latter risk, the risk of catastrophe, by the
American devotion to mastery as the *deus deorum*. Only
if we can bring out of the consulting room into the society,
as well as the ideas we have already brought out, the intelligent affection that contains and domesticates the otherwise threatening possibilities of insight, only if we can
institutionalize this intelligent affection in public life,
revolutionizing other institutions in the process if necessary, can we hope to call out the forces of life rather than
tap upon the door of death's angel.

The Freudian Ethic—No Guilt, No Responsibility

O. HOBART MOWRER

A^S WE move forward, with ever-accelerating tempo, into what we are pleased to call the Age of Science, we are faced by an awesome paradox. As man, through science, acquires more and more control over the external world, he has come to feel less and less capable of controlling himself, less and less the master of his own soul and destiny. In the same decade in which we produced the atomic submarine and started probing interstellar space, we have also seen, significantly, the emergence of the beatnik; personality disintegration has become endemic; and society itself is commonly said to be "sick." We remain optimistic about what man can continue to do through science by way of dealing with his environment, but we have become extremely pessimistic about man.

This reciprocal relationship is not accidental: the same presuppositions and intellectual operations that have given us such unprecedented power over nature when extended to ourselves produce a pervasive feeling of helplessness, confusion, resignation, desperation. We seem to be the hapless pawns of a great mechanical, impersonal juggernaut called the cosmos. By the very principles and premises that have led to the conquest of the outer world, we ourselves lose our autonomy, dignity, self-mastery, responsibility, indeed, our very identity. Little wonder, then, that we feel weak, lost, fearful, "beat." Being part of nature, we, too, apparently obey strict cause-and-effect principles; and if this be true, if our own experience and conduct are as rigidly determined and predetermined as is the rest of nature — the whole notion of purpose, responsibility, meaning seems to vanish. At the moment of our greatest technological triumphs, which include the tapping of almost unlimited sources of physical energy and the achievement of fabulous mechanical, chemical, and biological know-how, we become uncertain, lose confidence, and brood about annihilation. At the same time, some highly pertinent developments are quietly and unobtrusively occurring in psychological and sociological thought which hold promise of delivering us from our current predicament, both philosophically and practically.

Pre-Reformation Catholicism held man "doubly responsible," which is to say, capable of both good and evil. When, in this context, one behaved badly, it was to his discredit; and when one behaved well, it was decidedly to his credit. There was thus for each individual a sort of moral balance sheet, as it has been called, and ultimate salvation or damnation depended, quite simply and directly, on the number and magnitude of the entries on the two sides of this fateful ledger.

Obviously there was much in common sense and everyday experience to support such an ethical system, but there were also, unfortunately, broad opportunity and temptation for those responsible for its administration to pervert and abuse it. The problem of justice in *this* life presents difficulties enough, and when one enters into the subtleties of a life to come, the only restraints upon dogmatic assertion and egregious exploitation are the fertility of ecclesiastical imagination and the credulity of the faithful. For at least four hundred years prior to the Reformation, the will to resist such perversity had continued to decline, and by the beginning of the sixteenth century, the great triumphant Church Universal was fairly riddled with connivance, sophistry, sloth, and extortion.

Men of learning and independence of thought were, of course, well aware of this sad state of affairs long before the outbreak of what we think of as the Reformation proper. And pre-eminent among such men was the Dutch scholar and humanist Desiderius Erasmus, who made a two-pronged attack upon the situation. In his immediately successful and popular book *In Praise of Folly* (1511), he focused a delicate but deadly wit upon the Church's hypocrisy and corruption, and behind his Greek edition of the New Testament (1516) was the momentous imputation that it was not the Church that was the ultimate authority in religious matters but the Bible itself.

When, in 1517, Martin Luther nailed the ninety-five theses to the door of the Castle Church of Wittenberg, it was therefore not surprising that Erasmus was interested. The essence of Luther's position, particularly as it has filtered down to us through John Calvin and other Protestant expositors, is that man is responsible, so to say, in only one direction: capable of choosing the wrong and fully accountable for having done so, he is, however, supposedly unable to do anything whatever toward his own redemption and must wait, helplessly, upon the unpredictable favor, or "grace," of God. It is, of course, not difficult to see why such a curious and one-sided doctrine was conceived and advocated with such insistence: it cut the whole logic from under the Church's emphasis upon good works, including both penances and indulgences, and thus succeeded where more moderate programs of reform had failed.

Erasmus (in the tradition of the Apostle James, Pelagius, Jerome, and later, Arminius) had insisted upon human freedom and responsibility in the matter of both evil and good and had asked only for greater honesty in the assignment of the credit for each kind of action. But Luther and Calvin, seizing upon selected segments in the teachings of Saint Paul and Saint Augustine, stridently repudiated this position, and in so doing were able to produce an ideological and institutional change of enormous historical significance.

We are no doubt justified in looking back upon the Reformation as representing, in many ways, a magnificent achievement. But we have been slow to appreciate, it seems, how dearly it has cost us. Protestantism, whatever its virtues and strengths, has also had the tragic consequence of leaving us without clear and effective means of dealing with personal guilt. And it is this fact, I submit, more than any other that is responsible for what Paul Tillich has aptly called "the psychic disintegration of the masses" in modern times.

By 1900, the influence of religion and moral suasion had so far declined that the medical profession was being inundated by a new type of illness. Purely functional in origin but often expressed somatically, the new malady was characterized by a pervasive "loss of nerve," which, as a matter of medical convenience, was dubbed "neurosis." But the condition needed more than a name; it called for specific treatment, which medicine tried, without success, to provide. Hydrotherapy, hypnotism, electrical massage, bromides, and a dozen other nostrums came and went, but neurosis remained, unfathomed and unconquered.

In this era of confusion and crisis, psychoanalysis had its inception and spectacular proliferation. Religion had disqualified itself for dealing honestly and effectively with man's deepest moral and spiritual anguish. Freud's discoveries purported to rescue man from the perplexities of the Protestant ethic and the ravages of unresolved guilt, not by restoring him to full ethical responsibility but by relieving him of all responsibility. In short, the notion was that one should not feel guilty about anything. Freud tacitly agreed with Luther and Calvin that man is helpless to save (cure) himself, but he took the momentous further step of also holding no one accountable for having fallen into "neurosis" — which is just a medical euphemism for what had formerly been known as a state of sin — in the first place. "All behavior is caused" became the sanctimonious rallying cry for the new movement, for at one stroke it gave the appearance of advancing the science of mind and providing a powerful therapeutic procedure. Now, instead of mistreating the criminal, the insane, and the neurotic, we would understand and help them, treat them (for a fee). And this was all to be achieved not by a return to the outmoded principle of double responsibility but by adoption of a new and radical doctrine of double *irresponsibility*.

This innovation was, of course, acclaimed as a great scientific and cultural gain. Not only would we now be able to turn to others for treatment, thus confirming the Protestant thesis that we cannot help ourselves; we could also hold others accountable for our having got into such a predicament in the first place.

But as the clock of history has ticked off the decades of this century, we have gradually discovered that Freud's great postulate, not of total depravity but of total determinism, has liberated us only in the sense of dumping us from the frying pan into the fire. At long last we seem to be waking up to the fact that to be "free" in the sense of embracing the doctrine of double irresponsibility is not to be free at all, humanly speaking, but lost.

Within the past five years there has been a growing realization, at least in the disciplines most intimately concerned with such matters, of the futility, the deadly peril of this general trend. After an extensive study of the therapeutic claims and accomplishments of psychoanalysis, the English psychologist Dr. Hans Eysenck summed up the situation with this laconic statement: "The success of the Freudian revolution seemed complete. Only one thing went wrong: *the patients did not get any better.*" And this verdict has been amply borne out by numerous other inquiries of a similar kind.

Naturally, the doctrine of total determinism radiated from the field of psychopathology to criminology, and we were soon being told that not even those individuals convicted of legal crimes were really responsible; instead, they too were sick and in need of treatment rather than correction or conversion. Lawyers, judges, legislators, and psychiatrists are at present deeply embroiled in the question of criminal responsibility versus the doctrine of the irresistible impulse, but there have been several developments which suggest that the status of "expert testimony" may be undergoing serious reappraisal. The psychoanalytically oriented physician or psychiatrist who argues the doctrine of psychic determinism for others must either consistently apply it — and render himself irresponsible, incompetent, sick — or else assume an aura of omnipotence. The position of the psychiatric expert in our courts is currently not an enviable one.

A few years ago, Professor Richard La Piere of the Department of Sociology of Stanford University published a sobering volume with the tongue-in-cheek title *The Freudian Ethic*, in which he holds that in generally abandoning the Protestant ethic, whatever its shortcomings (and they are grievous), and espousing psychoanalysis we have moved, as an entire society, not toward salvation but perdition. With many other social analysts, La Piere agrees that, as a people, we are indeed sick, but argues that the very essence of our sickness is that we so freely resort to this concept instead of holding ourselves and others accountable.

While psychoanalysis was developing as a predominantly medical enterprise, a parallel movement with similar philosophic and practical implications was also taking form and gaining momentum in academic circles. I refer to the radical repudiation, in the first two or three decades of this century, of all that was inward, subjective, and personal, known as behaviorism, with its new and exclusive emphasis upon that form of cause-effect relationship implied by the so-called stimulus-response, or S-R, formula. Here determinism, although couched in somewhat different terms, was no less absolute than in psychoanalysis, and the individual was again relieved — or should we say deprived? — of all semblance of accountability. Behavior or action or conduct was the inevitable consequence of "antecedent stimulus conditions" (causes), and moral accountability became, in this context, a meaningless and, indeed, opprobrious concept. The conditioned and unconditioned reflex, in the language of Ivan Pavlov and J. B. Watson, was the "functional unit" of all behavior; and E. L. Thorndike, in his slightly different theory of habit, likewise spoke of stimulus-response "connections" or "bonds." All of which had at least the incidental effect, if not intent, of obliterating the whole notion of freedom, choice, responsibility by reducing behavior, absolutely and completely, to S-R connections and reflexes.

Some years ago the ambiguity of this situation came home to me in a particularly dramatic way. At that time I was still trying to do a little psychotherapy of the conventional kind, and on more than one occasion graduate students came to me for help who, in the course of our interviews, spontaneously remarked that one of the main inducements for them to go into psychology as a vocation was that they had long suffered from unresolved guilt, which psychology, with its scientific emphasis upon stimulus-response, cause-effect connections, seemed logically to eliminate. But the fact that these students were now in therapy was palpable proof that this stratagem had not worked. The behavioristic doctrine of total determinism manifestly does not deliver us from the one-sided determinism of Luther and Calvin any more effectively than does that brand of complete irresponsibility adduced by Freud. If the doctrines of Luther and Calvin disposed the Western world to "Christian despair," those of Freud and Watson have, it seems, engulfed us in a despair that is infinitely deeper.

It is only within the last decade or so that we have begun to see a way out. The existentialists, in their very legitimate protests against the general abrogation of responsibility — first one-sidedly, in Protestant theology, and then more systematically, in psychoanalysis and behaviorism — have recently been attracting some well-deserved attention. But when they go on to reject the scientific approach, totally and inherently, they are on dangerous ground and may shortly find themselves, in this regard, discredited.

Having denounced Protestant predestination and psychological determinism alike, what do the existentialists offer, alternatively? Only a counsel of brave despair, an admonition to have the courage to be, on the assumption that being (existence) *is* an ironic joke and ultimate tragedy. Just how do we come by this courage? By lifting ourselves by our own bootstraps? In practice, it seems that this philosophy leaves us quite as helpless and hopeless as does the Protestant principle, with its emphasis upon man's inevitable guilt and God's uncertain grace.

If one takes the time to examine contemporary behavior theory, one finds that scientific developments in psychology have moved a long way from the naïve and primitive assumptions of behaviorism. Now it is generally agreed that there is by no means a reflexive or ineluctable connection between stimulation and response. Now we are quite certain that the coupling between our sensory receptors and our muscles is much looser and infinitely more complicated than the earlier theories implied. According to present views, stimulation may suggest a given response or course of action, but whether we "give consent," as Catholic theologians would say, to the suggestion, thought, or image is dependent upon the hopes and fears which we weigh and ponder in deciding whether to act or refrain from acting. In other words, given a stimulus, a particular and predetermined response does not automatically pop out of the organism, as our earlier, push-button psychology seemed to demand. Response — and responsibility — in this new frame of reference is crucially dependent upon the anticipated consequences of our actions. In short, we have rediscovered reason. Instead of being merely stimulated (the Latin term for "goaded"), living organisms become goal-directed, purposive, deliberate, or, if you will, free and responsible.

Beginning with the naïve and oversimplified behaviorism of Watson, academic psychology in this century has thus achieved a relatively advanced degree of sophistication; whereas psychoanalysis, which started with Freud's highly elaborated and ingenious speculations, has rather steadily involuted, regressed. The original emphasis on unconscious (irresponsible) motivation has, of late years, given way to a new accent on "ego psychology," which involves frequent reference to "ego strength" and "ego weakness" in a manner unmistakably reminiscent of the older notions of character and will power; and with the ink hardly dry on this ego psychology literature, psychoanalysts are now beginning to show a new respect for and interest in the superego, or conscience.

These developments, I say, are retrogressive as far as Freud's original formulations go, but in terms of common sense they are decidedly in the right direction. However, they are suicidal as far as psychoanalysis itself is concerned, which was conceived and laid its claim to recognition as an independent discipline along very different lines.

All the developments just reviewed thus strike a new note, or at least one that has considerable novelty for contemporary men and women. Once more we are coming to perceive man as pre-eminently a social creature, whose greatest and most devastating anguish is experienced not in physical pain or biological deprivation but when he feels alienated, disgraced, guilty, debased as a person. And the thrust of much current therapeutic effort is in the direction of trying to help such individuals recover their sociality, relatedness, community, identity.

Here, surely, is a promising meeting ground for psychology, psychiatry, and sociology and for much that is common to both classical Judaism and authentic Christianity. But, logically and programmatically, it strikes at the heart of the Protestant principle. Yesterday, as a Presbyterian, I attended church and heard the minister quote Reinhold Niebuhr, with approval, to the effect that "Christian faith is more profound than mere moral idealism," thus echoing the contempt which Protestantism has always had for the "merely moral man." And the preceding Sunday I heard another minister preach a fine "Reformation" sermon on the theme that "the fruit of grace is responsibility for action in the world"; that is, the theme that we are good because — and if — we are saved, not the reverse. Scientific and humanistic thought can never, I believe, come to terms with such hyperbole. The fact that Protestant theologians keep reverting in their sermons to the question of just what it means to be "saved by grace," rather than by works, suggests that they are themselves not quite certain.

As a psychologist, I have no competence to judge the effectiveness of religion in saving men's immortal souls, and, I confess, this is not my major interest. But I do maintain that religion has great potential for serving, and saving, men and women in this world which is not now being at all adequately realized. If, in the secular sciences, we have rediscovered something of the logic and conditions of responsible action, perhaps this will be an encouragement to the theologians themselves to take a more courageous and responsible position and quit hiding behind a preposterous piece of medieval sophistry.

The Freudian Ethic — Self-Help
Through Self-Knowledge

PHILIP RIEFF

————•—•————

IT WAS Freud who insisted that the analyst must be a veiled figure. In that way, Freud made himself available for therapeutic purposes; the patient saw in him that character, or tangle of characters, with which he was too deeply involved. The first analyst thus became, in a guarded way, whatever the patient needed to find in him — father, mother, brother, boss, competitor, latent lover, manifest object of hatred.

Into this intimate relation between doctor and patient are marched the unemployed emotions of the patient's life, in order that they may be sorted out and put in working order. Thus, the analyst gets to know the patient. In contrast, the patient learns to know himself through his therapeutic association with the analyst. Of the analyst he knows nothing except what he can imagine. From this imagining, and through the informed deference of his attention, the analyst learns much of what he wants to know about the patient. Yet Freud refused to realize that in the doctor-patient relation the therapist himself is an incalculable element, involved no less than his patient.

If the two mysteries manage somehow to communicate, they accomplish that joint and greater mystery, a cure.

What the analyst can be to a patient, a doctrine may be, at times, to a culture. In both cases, the main therapeutic factor is the transference. Like patients, cultures may purge themselves of an inner conflict, caused by lingering attachments to some old doctrine, by attaching themselves to a doctrine that is new and yet closely related to the old. Thus, the Russians have not ceased to be a religious people; their Marxism makes history redemptive, instead of Christ. But the motif of redemption — for which Americans have never found a place — remains. Quite without intention, Freudianism opened up a dead end in the American inner life, encouraging the replication of an old moral attitude and at the same time supplying an answer of denial. In psychoanalysis, the puritan temper found a way to disapprove of itself.

Because it is so personal and humane a procedure, Freudian psychiatry has exhibited all the classic stigmas of a movement — splinter groups, rivalries within the leadership, secret councils, front men and organization men, passionate friendships turning into equally passionate hatreds. Freudian psychiatrists have had good reason to reject the notion that they are a movement. Any rending of the public veil can lead to a rending of private veils, which might endanger, or at least further complicate, the therapeutic effort. For therapeutic reasons, psychoanalysis is an esoteric discipline. As a movement, psychoanalysis necessarily sought to cover up the intense warfare of personality which, as a therapy, it sought to expose.

Unlike scientists free of the prophetic urge, Freud was

not satisfied to work modestly along the lines laid down by scientific discipline: in a small company of researchers, chasing after collections of data with interpretations — and after interpretations with data. Psychoanalysis was valuable in theory, according to Freud, so far as it was successful in practice. It changed men's minds as it cured them. Freud felt compelled by the nature of his discoveries, which men had to resist, to be the leader not merely of a movement but of an embattled one; he planned for the future of that movement in terms that can fairly be called moral — even if not in defense of established moralities. "Some larger group" was needed, he decided, than the local societies of Freudians that had sprung up to spread his theory with its practice; he wanted such a large group "working for a practical ideal."

The size of Freud's pedagogic ambition comes through clearly in his motives for founding the movement as an international body. This was no simple strategy to develop some licensing procedure, in order to screen entrants into the profession. Indeed, the movement was not yet so professional, and when it became so, in the famous controversy about the function of the psychoanalyst without a medical degree, Freud found himself on the losing, less professionally oriented side.

Psychoanalysis is not libertarian. As Freud conceived it, his was a genuinely neutralist movement; more precisely, a movement offering a doctrine of maturity which might free the proper student of it from the compulsion to identify with any and all movements. Despite invitations to declare himself philosophically and otherwise, Freud remained a neutralist all his life. Psychoanalysis perfectly represents the neutralism of his character.

As psychoanalysis became more adaptable, the hidden

force of Freud's character operated through the discipline, detached from his person and yet revealed in the neutral appearance that every analyst must present to his patients and, indeed, to the world. Despite periods of weakness, in which he toyed with ideas of linking his movement with others, Freud saw the dangers inherent in any such alliances. "We must in any event keep our independence. . . . In the end we can come together with all the parallel sciences." But that end appeared then, as now, far off; nor is it more clear now than it was at the time he gave this advice to one of his followers just which sciences are parallel to psychoanalysis.

As a movement, psychoanalysis was fortunate enough to achieve a countertransference to America, that richest and yet, symbolically, most needy of all patients. To this symbolically impoverished culture, psychoanalysis brought not a new or compelling symbolism, but the next best thing: a way of analyzing symbols that is itself of symbolic (and, therefore, therapeutic) value. From being a movement, psychoanalysis became a profession, practical and immensely necessary. In America, the clinician found himself in a culture that considered itself a little crippled and broken. Freud's was the perfect doctrine to help a culture that no longer respected itself and yet had already rejected all the earlier, established alternatives. Moreover, there was something about Protestantism itself that made it ready, upon decline, for psychoanalysis.

For Protestant culture, it was Calvin, with his doctrine of predestination, who first turned all action into symptom. Only the most careful scrutiny of the outer actions could give even a hint of the inner condition, whether that be of grace or damnation. When Freud analyzed all actions symptomatically, he appealed chiefly to persons, trained and yet troubled, in just those cultures that had once been Calvinist, or otherwise rigorously ascetic. The therapeutic of the psychological age is successor to the ascetic of the religious age, with the economic man of the age of enlightenment (and capitalism) as a merely transitional type.

Continuously, in both ascetic and therapeutic cultures, there is an inclination to see symptoms everywhere — except, of course, that the symptoms point to different sources. In the age of psychological man, God's design and the hope of penetrating it may have vanished utterly, as, in fact, the Calvinist also discovered, often to his relief, that it had; nevertheless, there remains the passion, innominate from the decline of Calvinism to the rise of Freudianism, for acquiring some knowledge of one's personal destiny.

To the therapeutic of the mid-twentieth century, as to the ascetic of the Reformation movements, all destinies had become intensely personal and not at all communal. The way to this self-knowledge, which may be in itself saving, is to trace back a person's conduct from symptom to the inner conditions responsible for that symptom. In the religious period, the symptom was called sin, and the neurotic, a sinner, self-convicted. The task of the clergy was to make the sinner hopefully aware of his sin; the task of the analyst is to make the neurotic therapeutically aware of his neurosis.

Residues of the old attribution of sin cling to the modern and popular usage of the term "neurotic." Like his predecessor the sinner, the neurotic is most reluctant to admit his weakness. In fact, this failure to admit a fundamental weakness is the most obvious characteristic of the inner wrong which the sinner-neurotic commits against himself. Such failure was once called pride. The thankless task of old ministers and new psychoanalysts consists first in educating for that state of awareness from which a person can cope with his weakness.

A detailed admission of weakness is the beginning of emotional (or spiritual) strength, in both the ascetic and therapeutic traditions. It is not a condition easily admitted, for the weak one may consider himself strong, and only others, near him, may have to bear the burden of his weakness. In this sense, a family may be dominated by its weakest member, who, to the unanalytic eye, may appear strongest merely because he is the most aggressive or has succeeded otherwise in building his neurosis into his character.

In the culture to which psychological man is heir, there has been an acute sense of the weakness of human character but a diminished capacity to feel compassion for it. As the religious mitigations of weakness, built into the ascetic tradition, withered away, all that remained was a test of strength — successful action in the conduct of life. These mitigations, or devices of release from the tension of trying to be good or successful, remained operative in Catholic cultures. In consequence, psychoanalytic therapy never found as ready and receptive a public in those areas of Western culture that remained Catholic, or nonascetic.

Meanwhile, in those parts of the ascetic West that had lost their religious impetus, the contempt for weakness, inherent anyway in Calvinist doctrine, grew steadily more powerful. The individiual, caught in this hard, dying culture, tried to hide his sense of weakness, for he no longer felt a compelling explanation for it; nor could he use something in his system of worship to escape this now intensely personal fault (no longer attributable to divine decision). The culture, always guilt-ridden, was no longer guilt-releasing. Without the remedy of grace or good works, conscience became the seat of emotional weakness rather than the sign of moral strength.

For Freud, strength was the rare bonus, weakness the common return on experience. By indicating again the universality of weakness — and, moreover, by suggesting new remedies for it — Freud challenged the tough indifference of the old ascetic attitude, while, at the same time, strengthening individuals to continue living in what remains a culture dominated by goals set in the ascetic period. In his determination to help an individual function more adequately in a situation essentially competitive from the cradle to the grave, Freud tempered the rivalrous mood of contemporary social life without challenging its validity. He thought thus to teach man how to snatch some personal success in living out of the general failure.

As a way of transforming the ascetic temper, now crabbed and mainly negative, psychoanalysis is no empty cipher, no shadow of religious doctrine. On the contrary, it is a doctrine suitable to this postreligious age. Even the goals of ascetic effort are disappearing in an economy based on leisure. If the former ascetic is to continue to work hard and live well, he must do so without any aim in mind other than the therapy of action which is living itself. The work of the ascetic must become the play of the therapeutic; that is the moral economy about which spokesmen of the new type, such as David Riesman, are theorizing.

As Freud saw him, psychological man had to learn how

to accept life as if it were a game, earnestly played, with each player aware that in the beginning he is so unpracticed that the game must remain a series of errors and penalties. Yet, learning finally to be a strategist on his own behalf, psychological man could meet demands upon his energy and character quite as rigorous as those made during a time when he had a God on his side and the comfort of natural law instead of mere laws of nature.

There is something old-fashioned about the psychoanalytic movement; it is, in fact, although more subtly than ever before, a movement of self-help. For all the analyst can do is teach another how to become his own therapist, strong in the knowledge of his particular weakness. Freud insisted on this modesty of purpose, which many critics have viewed as an unwarranted pessimism. But the alternative to Freud's modesty is the optimism of a fresh religious sense of personal service to some object other than the self. Such therapies seemed to Freud to exploit the very weaknesses from which man suffered and for which they sought therapy in the first place. Doctrines of salvation are always therapeutic. In a culture no longer capable of inventing such doctrines, Freud proposed a therapy that did not try to charm the suffering out of humanity but only restored the capacity to endure living. For those no longer childlike enough to be charmed, a restoration of capacity is the one gift necessary and prior to any small giving of themselves.

I must emphasize that Freud condemned the religious repressions for instrumental reasons, because they were failing. Because religion could no longer compel character but only distract it, Freud dared suggest, in the name of science, a new ethical straightforwardness. Faith had become another form of anxiety. Despite his occasional protests about its neutrality and limited purposes, Freud hoped his own science would contribute in a major way to the working out of a more controllable and rational alternative to those imaginative systems of increasing anxiety that we call "religion."

The Rejection of the Insane

GREER WILLIAMS

———— •—•———

THE way society handles its psychotics, by putting them away in human dumps, has been the subject of repeated public scandal. Surely the American press, whatever its failures, has lived up to its responsibility in this instance. It has published millions of words about inhuman care of the mentally sick since Nellie Bly wrote "Ten Days in a Madhouse" for the New York *World* in 1888. Most of this writing has been predicated on the assumption that if the plight — the shameful, subhuman condition — of the chronically sick of mind who populate the back wards of state hospitals were well exposed, the public would rise up in moral indignation and bring about reform. But the public remains unmoved, or, when it does move, does not move far enough. The thing that appears to be missing is public and professional action commensurate with the size of the mental illness problem.

One of the most revealing disclosures in *Action for Mental Health,* the final report of the Joint Commission on Mental Illness and Health, published in 1961 by Basic Books, is that comparatively few of 277 state hospitals — probably no more than 20 per cent — have actively participated in the modern therapeutic trend toward humane, healing hospitals and clinics of easy access and easy exit, instead of locked, barred, prisonlike depositories of alienated and rejected human beings.

It is true, of course, that these institutions never have been quite the end of the road that has become fixed in the public's mind. Actually, the number of patients now discharged annually from mental hospitals exceeds the annual number of first admissions. Including in the total figure the accumulated load of old patients who remain stubbornly psychotic, the average state hospital discharges 30 per cent of its patients each year. The worst mental hospitals return to the community 40 to 50 per cent of the patients they treat for schizophrenia, the most serious of major mental illnesses; the best hospitals discharge 75 to 85 per cent.

But the typical state hospital, through the accumulation of its chronically ill patients and its tendency to make many patients worse instead of better, remains substantially what it was a hundred years ago, an asylum for the "incurably insane." As such, it is characterized by rigidly authoritarian control, solemn vigilance, and covert despair. It does a good job of keeping patients physically alive and mentally sick. If a patient will not eat, he may be force-fed; if he will not talk — well, he is less trouble that way. And as for the tranquilizing drugs, they make agitated patients friendlier and more cooperative, and therefore make the lives of attendants and nurses more tolerable. Thus, the drugs have introduced enthusiasm where there was none.

There has been some increase in hospital staffs. The average hospital has one employee (including psychiatrists) for every three patients; this compares with two or more employees per patient (not counting attending physicians) in the average community general hospital. But, with the exceptions indicated, the state hospital system of caring for the mentally ill — nearly a million patients every year — has shown an amazing resistance to change for the better.

What is wrong here? Why, in the care of the mentally ill, do we lag, in the achievement of both our humanitarian and scientific goals, behind the public demand for mental health services — especially in clinics, where the waiting lists run on for months, and even years — and behind other major public health programs?

The reason of longest standing, perhaps, is that people do not recognize the insane, or psychotic, simply as sick human beings in need of help. Instead, people see the psychotic's behavior, the symptoms of illness, as immoral or illegal, and therefore deserving of punishment rather than pity. We frequently go to great lengths to explain our friend's clearly irrational and uncontrolled behavior simply as "the way he is"; that is, we put up with him until he does something that brings him a mental patient or psycho label. After that, we do not quite trust him, whatever he does.

Publicly recorded insanity, like convicted crime, tends to produce a stigma that cuts the bonds of human fellowship. Many other dread diseases — tuberculosis, syphilis, cancer — have in their time and their way branded their victims as unfit for human society. In modern times, however, the horror and shame of diseases recognized to be physically caused and highly lethal have tended to disappear — or, at any rate, to be offset — as they came under public scrutiny and attack. The person who goes to the hospital with cancer or heart disease and recovers is accepted back into the community in a way that the mental patient almost never is.

The stigma question leads us to the feeling of helplessness and hopelessness that the insane produce in us. If we only knew what to do with a mentally ill person, how to manage him, where to take him, how to get him well again, we would not feel so confused. Even the family doctor, let alone the psychiatrist, is hard to reach these days. At best, the mentally ill are a great nuisance; at worst, we are scared to death of them. In either case, they embarrass us.

In a broad sense, what we are saying is that if we only had more scientific knowledge of diagnosis and treatment or preventive techniques at our disposal, then we could conquer mental illness, including our feelings about it. There is a mixture of truth and fallacy here. In the first place, the mentally ill on the whole are not as dangerous as most people believe. Those disposed to physical violence are the exception rather than the rule, although, as with airliners, we read more about the few crashes than all the safe landings. When attacked by a person bent on destruction, one must defend himself or flee. But often psychotics are enraged by an impetuous or treacherous use of force against them that would equally anger a normal person.

Second, mental illness is not categorically a one-way street. Nobody is totally insane, any more than he is totally infected with a germ or totally cancerous. Some get well without treatment; others improve greatly if treated well; some recover and have later relapses; a few never recover. It only misleads, therefore, to say that lack of an adequate technology, or a good scientific tool kit, is the main reason why the public fails to attack mental illness with vigor proportionate to the size of the problem.

Medical science is still searching for the cause and cure of cancer and of the major forms of heart disease, but the lack of better methods of treatment or prevention has not resulted in inhuman, substandard care for patients. In reality, the schizophrenic has a far better chance for recovery and a useful life than the victim of any of several major physical illnesses. There is an important economic difference, of course: in lung cancer or coronary thrombosis, death removes treatment failures from the scene, whereas chronic schizophrenics do not get well and do not die; they accumulate in public institutions.

Some would say that this is the big obstacle — so many patients with major mental illness live on and become indigent. Long hospitalization and psychiatric treatment impose costs the average family cannot afford. Thus, the burden of mental patient care, a good four fifths of it, falls on the state. State hospitals spend from two to six dollars per patient per day, compared with upward of thirty dollars a day in community general hospitals and leading private mental hospitals.

It is customary, at least among Republicans, automatically to regard state medicine as bad medicine, because it imposes a tax burden and involves politics. These make for a poor quality of medical care, it is argued. The generalization is a weak one, however. County tuberculosis hospitals have done a generally creditable job of long-term care for tuberculous patients at taxpayers' expense, at an average of thirteen dollars per patient per day. Many did so even before modern advances in surgical and drug treatment. Of course, the patient load has been smaller for tuberculosis than for mental illness.

The Veterans' Administration psychiatric hospitals, themselves well within the snake-pit range of description until after the war, now provide an acceptable quality of tax-paid mental patient care at an average cost per patient of twelve dollars per day. It is easy to document this observation. The hospitals' national standard-setting agency, the Joint Commission on Accreditation of Hospitals, has approved only 30 per cent of state hospitals, contrasted with 100 per cent of V.A. psychiatric hospitals. Why can't state hospitals do as well? One answer seems to be that the federal government has far greater financial resources than the states have, and, above all, veterans have influence through a well-organized pressure group.

We now approach the nub of the matter. The insane sick are friendless, unless their families have money or a mental health worker unexpectedly befriends them. It is a truism in voluntary health organizations that people are prone to work for a cause which they can identify with personally. But an organization which seeds itself with workers who have been mentally ill accepts a considerable handicap. And how many others are prepared to identify themselves with insanity in the family? One psychiatrist, Dr. J. Sanbourne Bockoven of Framingham, Massachusetts, pinpoints these issues: "The very essence of mental illness is an incapacity to get along with other people, hence organization behind a leader is impossible. The friends or relatives of the mentally ill are equally immobilized through fear of stigmatizing themselves."

Quite a number of groups of former mental patients have come into being and then languished; none has flourished as, for example, Alcoholics Anonymous has. The difference seems to be that alcoholics, basically neurotic, are usually successful persons while sober. In any event, their "cure," refusing a drink, is only slightly stigmatizing.

A psychosis is essentially a social disorder, or, as defined by the late Dr. Harry Stack Sullivan, founder of the Washington School of Psychiatry, one involving interpersonal relationships. The normal person will do whatever he has to do to get along in his group; the psychotic will not. He suffers from a sort of mental arthritis that turns individualism into a disease.

The person with an acute psychosis sooner or later disturbs or offends other people and is likely to be treated as a disturber and offender. He does not fit our conception of a sick person in need of help; often he does not recognize himself as sick. It has been observed countless times that the sight or even the thought of a person "out of his mind" stimulates fear in us; fear of what the irrational person might do, fear of what we ourselves might do in response to this threat, fear arising from the power of suggestion that "I, too, will go crazy." For many of us, self-control is a lifelong problem. The insane person has somehow lost control. We feel sorry for him, but not nearly as sorry as relieved to have him out of the way. We have some of the same feelings about a physically sick person, too, but he gives us little reason to lose faith in him. We can see that he is sick. If conscious, he knows he is sick. He behaves predictably.

If we spent our lives among psychotics rather than encountering them rarely, we would realize that a calm alertness is desirable, but fearfulness and distrust are not necessary. You hear of patients killing themselves, but did you ever hear of a patient killing his psychiatrist or nurse? It is extremely rare. It was known more than one hundred and fifty years ago by the French physician Philippe Pinel and the Quaker layman William Tuke that figuratively turning the other cheek is not only a humane but a healing approach to the insane if pursued with friendly firmness and the sane recognition that the first problem is breaking the vicious circle of provocation and retaliation. Of course, it takes a good deal more brotherly love and physical courage than many of us have to find this out.

The mental hygiene, or mental health, movement was born out of the need to relieve medical and social guilt over the unloving and often brutally punishing way mental hospital workers used to treat the uncooperative insane. Not a physician but a young layman, a manic-depressive college graduate named Clifford Beers, while still in a strait jacket and padded cell, swore he would get out and crusade against the evils he saw in mental institutions. Beers succeeded; his *A Mind That Found Itself* was published in 1908.

Perhaps today Beers would receive a place on the future-appointments book of a good psychiatrist, work out his hostility and aggressions on the couch, and pay the fee out of his Book-of-the-Month Club and Hollywood royalties. Happily, he won the support of three great doctors who gave him a hearing rather than a diagnosis: William James, the psychologist; Adolf Meyer, the psychiatrist, and William H. Welch, the pathologist. They, with others, founded the National Committee for Mental Hygiene and made Beers its executive secretary.

Almost from the outset the movement was enthralled with the vision of doing away with mental illness entirely. One of the original circle, probably Meyer, told Beers that his own illness could have been prevented. Was not that the better approach? It turned out to be wishful thinking, but the mental hygienists had their heads turned by the microbe hunters, who were having impressive successes in disease prevention through sanitation and immunization. Eugenics and progressive education were also in the air. The larger goal became "building healthy minds in healthy bodies," but instead of a simple remedy such as chlorine in drinking water or a vaccine to be scratched into the arm, there were complicated concepts of mental health education and child guidance. Yet raising a child for a mentally healthy maturity is still a matter of theory, not scientific predictability, a half century later, even when we add the interpretations and zeal of psychoanalysis. There is little scientific evidence today that mental hygiene education does in fact prevent mental illness, although we certainly believe it promotes human understanding and reduces stress. Furthermore, as our knowledge of genetic chemistry and the mathematical certainty of accidents of chromosome linkage has advanced, there is little cause for optimism about the production of healthy minds to order.

There are many persons in the mental health field, including some staff members of the National Institute of Mental Health, who still pursue the will-o'-the-wisp of positive mental health in preference to trying to love the mentally ill. Ironically, Beers himself provided some substance for their attitudes. His crusade did not come off well, in either its original or acquired objectives. As is characteristic of one with his disorder, he had his ups and downs, eventually dying in a mental hospital in 1943.

The medical profession is as remiss as the public itself in grappling with the mental illness problem. It is common knowledge, confirmed by surveys, that the average physician as well as the average layman has unfavorable, sometimes openly antagonistic attitudes toward persons with psychological disturbances and toward psychiatrists themselves. The ordinary doctor's training and experience is not slanted toward an appreciation of emotions and their implications, and many doctors have only one approach to mental illness: they try to get the patients out of their offices as quickly as possible.

Surprisingly enough, when we narrow the circle of rejection to the private practice of psychiatry, we find somewhat the same situation as far as psychotics are concerned. I have heard psychiatrists say they were interested in neurotics but wanted no part of psychotics. Their logic was indisputable: they could help the former but not the latter, they said; besides, their only possible basis for successful psychotherapy is that the patient wants help and will pay for it. Psychiatrists who work in mental hospitals or clinics with psychotics do not share these opinions; they frankly concede the limitations of psychiatric knowledge, but know and can see that persons with major mental illness can be helped, whether they pay or not. These psychiatrists are vastly in the minority.

Not long ago a young psychiatrist clarified for me the pivotal difficulty in the care of psychotics. I have the general impression that he had witnessed major mental illness in his own family, and therefore had the strongest of motives for wanting to help its victims — a personal one.

"Even before I went to medical school," he told me, "I wanted to go into psychiatry and I wanted to treat psychotics. This was the real challenge. So I came to Boston to train in a hospital under three men who had the same objective. When I finished, I received a teaching and research appointment in this hospital, but the salary was low and I had the privilege of doing part-time private practice if I wished.

"So I started seeing patients privately, and again decided to concentrate on psychotics. I reached a point where I was treating six, in intensive psychotherapy, and felt that I was rebuilding their characters. There is a great satisfaction in it, but I found that I simply could not take them — not continuously. These are the most trying, tiring people on earth. So I cut down to three psychotics and filled in the open time with neurotics and mild character disorders."

I felt a little sad, but also vastly relieved. Psychiatrists and their public relations spokesmen long have remonstrated with the public for turning its back on the mentally ill. "Mental illness is no different from any other illness. The mentally ill should be treated the same way as any other sick people." These are expressions of good intentions. The public gives them some lip service, and a few sensitive and compassionate persons succeed in living by these principles, but our actions show that most of us really don't agree with them, and for good reason. Psychotics are hard to take. Even the most conscientious of psychiatrists may find them so.

A study made at Washington University, St. Louis, of criminal psychopaths confirms the pervasiveness of this rejection mechanism. Among social scientists studying the antisocial character of these persons, there was reported to be an active but not readily admitted effort to escape working with them. Likewise, a study of chronic schizophrenic patients under experimental treatment with a certain hormone at McLean Hospital in Boston bears out our thesis. A scientific analysis indicated that the treated patients were having more normal social relationships with other patients than those receiving a placebo. Further analysis showed that the treated group was not initiating these friendly approaches, but that the other patients were approaching them. It is of interest that the apparent effect of the drug was to make its users somewhat more receptive.

The psychotic's lack of appeal strikes me as a satisfactory explanation of why, in the last analysis, the fight against mental illness never seems to get anywhere at the level of social action. It is safe to say that in our culture nobody gets anywhere without a positive appeal of some kind. However, upon further reflection, I would agree that the explanation is not a satisfactory one at the intellectual level. Why do we have so much difficulty in understanding psychological problems and solving them in the first place?

The great difficulty is that many people have trouble in recognizing psychological sickness as sickness, or in seeing sickness as having psychological forms. Unless the mind is educated to think in psychological as well as physical terms from a fairly early age, it may experience great difficulty in later life in thinking about itself and about other minds in relation to itself. The difficulty can be overcome, but against some odds, for the mind seems to resist the process, as if, in the varied universe of knowing, it were the one constant — fixed, dependable, *sane*. Most of us, in sum, are psychologically handicapped persons, mentally blind to our physical bias.

The mental health movement is engaged in an uphill pull against intellectual resistance to psychological insight. The nature of the psychotic's trouble impels him to reject social order, and, heeding the ancient law of retaliation, we repay him in kind.

There is some evidence that the process has begun to reverse itself among younger, better educated people, since we have had a two-generation exposure to psychological and psychoanalytic information. Therapeutic techniques have evolved that break the circle of rejection and defeat it. Evaluations of the psychosocial approaches, proving old truths scientifically, show that some psychiatrists get amazingly good results from psychotherapy with schizophrenics. They also show that other persons, working individually or in groups in hospitals and clinics — social workers, psychologists, nurses, occupational therapists, attendants, enlightened volunteers — can do as much for the psychotic in their way as the psychiatrist can in his (it may be in the same way). In all cases, some kind of as yet ill-defined personal relationship develops between the therapist and patient. In most cases, the secret of reducing the fears, frustrations, and fatigues that beset those who try to work with psychotics is close moral support, given regularly or as needed by the therapist's superiors or peers.

We know that insanity presents a quite different problem from a broken leg or gallbladder attack. We also know that the line between abnormal and normal behavior is so blurred that anyone may step across it at one time or another. The psychotic, like the normal person, has good days as well as bad. The difference between mental illness and mental health is not as zero to a hundred, but, to press a fictitious measurement, it may perhaps be as little as forty-nine to fifty-one.

Consequently, with a fuller awareness of what people understand and believe, the mental health educators are going to have to revise their mental hygiene copybooks. Mental health is different from other health problems.

Because it is different, we have to solve it differently. This new approach remains to be tested and proved, of course. Nevertheless, the older one has left so much to be desired, as studies of public attitudes have abundantly shown, that we have nothing to lose through a sharper public focus on our resistance to thinking about mental illness and on our rejection of its victims. We can hardly hope to hit a target unless we can locate it and aim at it.

PART III

Psychiatry and Culture

The Language of Pundits

ALFRED KAZIN

—•—

IT IS curious that Freud, the founder of psychoanalysis, remains the only first-class writer identified with
the psychoanalytic movement. It was, of course, Freud's
remarkable literary abilities that gave currency to his
once difficult and even "bestial" ideas; it was the insight
he showed into concrete human problems, the discoveries
whose force is revealed to us in a language supple, dramatic, and charged with excitement of Freud's mission as
a "conquistador" into realms hitherto closed to scientific
inquiry, that excited and persuaded so many readers of
his books. Even the reader who does not accept all of
Freud's reasoning is aware, as he reads his interpretation
of dreams, of the horror associated with incest, of the
Egyptian origins of Moses, that this is a writer who is bent
on making the most mysterious and unmentionable matters entirely clear to himself, and that this fundamental
concern to get at the truth makes dramatis personae out of
his symbols and dramatic episodes out of the archetypal
human struggles he has described. It is certainly possible
to read Freud, even to enjoy his books, without being convinced by him, but anyone sensitive to the nuances and
playfulness of literary style, to the shaping power of a

great intellectual conception, is not likely to miss in Freud
the peculiar urgency of the great writer; for myself, I can
never read him without carrying away a deeply engraved,
an unforgettable sense of the force of human desire.

By contrast, many of the analysts who turn to writing
seem to me not so much writers as people clutching at a
few ideas. Whenever I immerse myself, very briefly, in
the magisterial clumsiness of Dr. Gregory Zilboorg, or
the slovenly looseness of Dr. Theodore Reik, or the tensely
inarticulate essays of Dr. Harry Stack Sullivan, or the
purringly complacent formulas of Dr. Edmund Bergler,
or even the smoothly professional pages of Dr. Erich
Fromm, I have a mental picture of a man leaping up from
his chair, crying with exultation, "I have it! The reason
for frigidity in the middle-aged female is the claustropho-
bic constitution!", and straightway rushing to his publisher. Where Freud really tried to give an explanation to
himself of one specific human difficulty after another,
and then in his old-fashioned way tried to show the determination of one new fact on another, it is enough these
days for Dr. Bergler to assert why all writers are blocked,
or for Dr. Theodore Reik, in his long-winded and inconse-
quential trek into love and lust, to announce that male
and female are so different as to be virtually of different
species. The vital difference between a writer and someone who merely is published is that the writer seems always to be saying to himself, as Stendhal actually did,
"If I am not clear, the world around me collapses." In a
very real sense, the writer writes in order to teach himself, to understand himself, to satisfy himself; the publishing of his ideas, though it brings gratifications, is a
curious anticlimax.

Of course, there are psychoanalyst-writers who aim at

understanding for themselves, but don't succeed. Even in Freud's immediate circle, several of the original disciples, having obtained their system from the master, devoted themselves to specialties and obsessions that, even if they were more than private *idées fixes*, like Otto Rank's belief in the "birth trauma," were simply not given the hard and lucid expression necessary to convince the world of their objectivity. Lacking Freud's striking combination of intellectual zeal and common sense, his balanced and often rueful sense of the total image presented by the human person, these disciples wrote as if they could draw upon Freud's system while expanding one or two favorite notions out of keeping with the rest. But so strongly is Freud's general conception the product of his literary ability, so much is it held together only in Freud's own books, by the force of his own mind, that it is extraordinary how, apart from Freud, Freudianism loses its general interest and often becomes merely an excuse for wild-goose chases.

Obviously these private concerns were far more important to certain people in Freud's own circle than was the validity of Freudianism itself. When it came to a conflict between Freudianism and their own causes (Otto Rank) or their desire to be uninhibited in mystical indefiniteness (C. G. Jung), the body of ideas which they had inherited, not earned, no longer existed for them. Quite apart from his personal disposition to remain in control of the movement which he had founded, Freud was objectively right in warning disciples like Ferenczi, Rank, Adler, and Stekel not to break away from his authority. For the analyst's interest in psychoanalysis is likely to have its origin in some personal anxiety, and some particularly unstable people (of whom there were several in Freud's circle), lacking Freud's unusual ability not only to work through his own neuroses but to sublimate everything into the grand creative exultation of founding a movement, committed themselves fruitlessly to the development of their unsystematic ideas, found it impossible to heal themselves by the *ad hoc* doctrines they had advanced for this purpose, and even relapsed into serious mental illness and suicide.

Until fairly recently, it was perfectly possible for anyone with a Ph.D. (in literature or Zen or philology) to be a "psychotherapist" in New York state. I have known several such therapists among the intellectuals of New York, and I distinguish them very sharply from the many skillful and devoted lay analysts, with a direct training in psychoanalysis, who are likely to have an objective concern with the malady of their patients. The intellectuals with Ph.D.s who transferred from other professions to the practice of psychoanalysis still seem to me an extreme and sinister example of the tendency of psychoanalysis to throw up the pundit as a type. Like modern intellectuals everywhere, intellectuals as self-made analysts are likely to have one or two ruling ideas which bear obvious relation to their private history, but which, unlike intellectuals generally, they have been able to impose upon people who came to them desperately eager for orientation in their difficulties. In short, the ruling weakness of intellectuals, which is to flit from idea to idea in the hope of finding some instrument of personal or world salvation, has often become a method of indoctrination. All the great figures in psychoanalysis have been egotists of the most extreme sort; all the creative ones, from Freud himself to the late unfortunate Dr. Wilhelm Reich, were openly ex-

asperated with the necessity of having to deal with patients at all. They were interested only in high thinking,
though Freud at least tempered his impatience enough to
learn from his patients; the objective power, the need to
examine symptoms in others, never left him.

By contrast, the intellectual who is looking for an audience or a disciple has often, as a psychotherapist, found
one in his patient. And the obvious danger of exploiting
the credulous, the submissive, the troubled (as someone
said, it is the analyst's love that cures the patient, and certain intellectuals love no one so much as a good listener),
which starts from a doctrine held by the analyst in good
faith but which may be no less narrow-minded or fanati-
cal for all that, seems to me only an extension of the passion for explaining everything by psychoanalysis which
literary intellectuals have indulged in so long. When I
think of some of the intellectuals who have offered their
services as therapists, I cannot but believe that to them
the patient is irrelevant to their own passion for intellectual indoctrination. My proof of this is the way they write.
Ever since Freud gave the word to so many people less
talented than himself, it has become increasingly clear
that whatever psychoanalysis may have done for many
troubled people, it has encouraged nonwriters to become
bad writers and mediocre writers to affect the style of
pundits. For the root of all bad writing is to be distracted,
to be self-conscious, not to have your eye on the ball, not
to confront a subject with entire directness, with entire
humility, and with concentrated passion. The root of all
bad writing is to compose what you have not worked out,
de haut en bas, for yourself. Unless words come into the
writer's mind as fresh coinages for what the writer him-

self knows that he knows, knows to be true, it is impossible for him to give back in words that direct quality of experience which is the essence of literature.

Now, behind the immense power and authority of psychoanalytical doctrines over contemporary literature — which expresses itself in the motivation of characters, the images of poetry, the symbol hunting of critics, the immense congregation of psychiatric situations and of psychiatrists in contemporary plays and novels — lies the urgent conviction, born with modern literature in the Romantic period, the seedbed of Freudian ideas, that literature can give us knowledge. The Romantic poets believed in the supremacy of imagination over logic exactly as we now believe that the unconscious has stories to tell which ordinary consciousness knows nothing of. And just as the analyst looks to free association on the part of the patient to reveal conflicts buried too deep in the psyche to be revealed to the ordinarily conscious mind, so the Romantic poets believed that what has been buried in us, far from the prying disapprovals of culture, stands for "nature," our true human nature. A new world had been revealed to the Romantics, a world accessible through the imagination that creates art. And Freud, who also felt that he had come upon a new world, said that his insights had been anticipated by literary men in particular; he felt that he had confirmed, as scientific doctrine, profound discoveries about our buried, our archetypal, our passionate human nature that philosophers and poets had made as artists.

Had made as artists. Nietzsche, who also anticipated many of Freud's psychological insights, said that Dostoevski was the only psychologist who had ever taught him anything. No doubt he meant that the characters Dostoevski had created, the freshness of Dostoevski's perceptions, the powerful but ironic rationality of Dostoevski's style had created new facts for him to think of in comparison with the stale medical formulas of psychiatry in his time. Similarly, Freud said of Dostoevski that "before genius analysis lays down its arms," indicating that with the shaping power of the artist who can create characters like old Karamazov and Prince Myshkin, with the genius that in its gift of creation actually parallels life instead of merely commenting on it, analysis cannot compete. And in point of fact we do learn more about the human heart from a stupendous creation like the Karamazov family than we ever do from all the formulatic "motivations" of human nature. Just as each human being, in his uniqueness, escapes all the dry formulas and explanations about human nature, so a great new creation in imaginative literature, a direct vision of the eternal like William Blake's or an unprecedented and unassimilable human being like old Karamazov, automatically upsets and rearranges our hardened conceptions of human nature.

There is no substitute for life, for the direct impression of life; there is no deep truth about life, such as writers bring home to us, that does not come in the form of more life. To anyone who really knows how rare and precious imaginative creation is — how small, after all, is that procession which includes Dante's Paolo and Francesca, Shakespeare's Othello, and Tolstoy's Natasha — how infinitely real in suggestion is the character that has been created in and through imagination, there is something finally unbearable, the very opposite of what literature is for, in the kind of metallic writing which now so often serves in a novel to "motivate" a character.

Maybe the only tenable literary role which novelists and poets, as well as critics and psychologists, now want to play is that of the expert — the explainer, the commentator, the analyst. Just as so many psychoanalysts want to be writers, so many writers now want to be analysts. And whenever I rise up at intervals from my dutiful immersion in certain specimens of contemporary literature, I find it hard to say who has less to contribute to literature, the psychiatrist who wants to push a few small ideas into a book or the novelist who in the course of a story breaks down into writing like a psychoanalyst.

The deterioration of language in contemporary fiction into the language of pundits is not often noticed by critics — perhaps because the novelists have taken to writing like critics. But it is by no means the highbrow or intellectual novelist, like Mary McCarthy, who in a single story for *Partisan Review* is likely to produce so many deliberate symbols, who is the only offender against art. John O'Hara, in *From the Terrace*, wrote of the mother of his hero that "What had happened to her was that she unconsciously abandoned the public virginity and, again unconsciously, began to function as a woman." Of the Eaton brothers, O'Hara made it clear that "If William slapped Alfred or otherwise punished him, the difference in ages was always mentioned while William himself was being punished; and each time that that occurred the age separation contributed to a strengthening of the separation that was already there because of, among other considerations, the two distinct personalities." This is a novelist? Frankly, I have the impression that many of the younger novelists have learned to write fiction from reading the new critics, the anthropologists and psychologists. I cannot begin to enumerate all the novels of recent years, from Ralph Ellison's *Invisible Man* to Vance Bourjaily's recent *Confessions of a Spent Youth,* which describe American social customs, from college up, as fulfilling the prescription of tribal rites laid down by the anthropologists. But whereas an angry and powerful novelist, as Ellison was in *Invisible Man,* whatever helpful hints he may get from psychiatrically oriented literary critics, will aim at the strongest possible image of Negro suffering and confusion in a hostile society, Van Bourjaily, in his recent novel, has his hero preface his description of a business smoker by apologizing that "it would take the calm mind of an anthropologist to describe objectively the rites with which the advertising tribe sent its bachelor to meet his bride."

I don't know what repels me more in such writing, the low spirits behind such prosiness or the attempted irony that is meant to disguise the fact that the writer is simply not facing his subject directly but is looking for something to say about it. No wonder that a passage like this sounds not like fiction but a case history: "I had a good time with Vicky during those two or three months; at the same time, I was learning about the social structure of the town and that of the school which, with certain exceptions for unusual individuals, reflected it; Vicky was more or less middle middle. As a friend of hers, since my own status was ambiguous, it seemed to me that I must acquire hers by association." And Mr. Bourjaily's book *is* a case history, though so meanderingly self-absorbed, for the most part, that it comes splendidly alive when the hero describes a visit to his relatives in the Near East; for a few pages we are onto people whom Mr. Bourjaily has to describe for us, since they are new types, and then we get free of the motivational analysis that is the novelist's desperate response to people who he thinks are too familiar to be conveyed directly. This is a curious idea of a novel — as if it were the subject, rather than the point of view, which made it boring.

The true writer starts from autobiography, but he does not end there; and it is not himself he is interested in, but the use he can make of self as a literary creation. Of course, it is not the autobiographical subject that makes such books as Mr. Bourjaily's flat; it is the relatively shallow level from which the author regards his own experience. The mark of this is that the writer does not even bother to turn his hero into a character; he is just a focus for the usual "ironic" psychological comment. If the writer nowadays sees himself as a pundit, he sees his hero as a patient. What, in fact, one sees in many contemporary American novelists today is the author as analyst confronting his alter ego as analysand. The novel, in short, becomes simply an instrument of self-analysis, which may be privately good for the writer (I doubt it) but is certainly boring to his readers.

The deterioration of language in contemporary "imaginative" literature — this reduction of experience to flat, vaguely orphic loose statements — seems to me most serious whenever, in our psychiatrically centered culture, spontaneity becomes an arbitrary gesture which people can simulate. Among the Beat writers, spontaneity becomes a necessary convention of mental health, a way of simulating vitality, directness, rough informality, when in fact the literary works produced for this pose have no vitality, are not about anything very significant, and are about as rough as men ever are using dirty words when they cut themselves shaving. The critic Harold Rosenberg once referred scathingly to the "herd of independent minds"; when I read the Beat and spontaneous poets en bloc, as I have just done in Donald Allen's anthology of the "new" American poetry, I feel that I am watching a bunch of lonely Pagliaccis making themselves up to look gay. To be spontaneous on purpose, spontaneous all the time, spontaneous on demand is bad enough; you are obeying not yourself but some psychiatric commandment. But to convert this artificial, constant, unreal spontaneity into poetry as a way of avoiding the risks and obligations of an objective literary work is first to make a howling clown out of yourself and then deliberately to cry up your bad literature as the only good literature.

The idea of the Beat poets is to write so quickly that they will not have to stand up for the poem itself; it is enough to be caught in the act of writing. The emphasis is not on the poem but on themselves being glimpsed in the act of creation. In short, they are functioning, they are getting out of the prison house of neurosis, they are positive and free. "Look, Ma, no hands!" More than this, they are shown in the act of writing poems which describe them in the act of living, just about to write poems. *"Morning again, nothing has to be done/ maybe buy a piano or make fudge/ At least clean the room up, for sure like my farther/ I've done flick the ashes & buts over the bedside on the floor."* This is Peter Orlovsky, "Second Poem."

Elsewhere, the hysterical demand for spontaneity as an absolute value means that everything in the normal social world becomes an enemy of your freedom. You want to destroy it so as to find an image of the ecstasy that has become the only image of reality the isolated mind will settle for. It is a wish for the apocalypse that lies behind the continued self-righteous muttering that the world is about to blow up. The world is not about to blow up, but behind the extreme literary pose that every-thing exists to stifle and suppress and exterminate us per-haps lies the belief, as Henry Miller plainly put it in *Tropic of Cancer*, that "For a hundred years or more the world, *our* world, has been dying. . . . The world is rotting away, dying piecemeal. But it needs the *coup de grâce*, it needs to be blown to smithereens. . . . We are going to put it down — the evolution of this world which has died but which has not been buried. We are swimming on the face of time and all else has drowned, is drowning, or will drown."

The setting of this apocalyptic wish is the stated enmity between the self and the world, between the literary imagi-nation and mere reality — a tension which was set up by Romanticism and which Freudianism has sharpened and intensified to the point where the extreme Romantic, the Beat writer, confesses that the world must be destroyed in order that the freedom of his imagination proceed to its infinite goal. Romanticism put so much emphasis on the personal consciousness that eventually the single person came to consider himself prior to the world and, in a sense, replacing it; under Romanticism, the self aban-doned its natural ties to society and nature and empha-sized the will. The more the single conscious mind saw the world as an object for it to study, the more conscious-ness was thrown back on itself in fearful isolation; the individual, alone now with his consciousness, preoccu-pied in regarding himself and studying himself, had to exercise by more and more urgent exertions of will that relationship to the world which made consciousness the emperor of all it could survey — the world was merely raw material to the inquiring mind.

Freud, himself a highly conservative and skeptical

thinker with a deeply classical bias in favor of limitation, restraint, and control, could not have anticipated that his critique of repression, of the admired self-control of the bourgeoisie, would in time, with the bankruptcy of bourgeois values, become a philosophy for many of his followers. Freudianism is a critique of Victorian culture; it is not a prescription for living in the twentieth century, in a world where the individual finds himself increasingly alienated from the society to which he is physically tied. Freud once wrote in a letter to Romain Rolland: "Psychoanalysis also has its scale of values, but its sole aim is the enhanced harmony of the ego, which is expected successfully to mediate between the claims of the instinctual life [the id] and those of the external world; thus between inner and outer reality.

"We seem to diverge rather far in the role we assign to intuition. Your mystics rely on it to teach them how to solve the riddle of the universe; we believe that it cannot reveal to us anything but primitive, instinctual impulses and attitudes . . . worthless for orientation in the alien, external world."

It was the Romantics who handed down to modern writers the necessity to think of the world as "alien and external." By now so many writers mechanically think of it this way that it is no wonder that they look for a philosophy of life to the "primitive, instinctual impulses and attitudes," though, as Freud knew, they are "worthless for orientation in the alien, external world." Man cannot cheat his own mind; he cannot bypass the centrality of his own intelligence. Yet is not sole reliance on the "primitive, instinctual impulses" exactly the *raison d'être* of so many Beat poems and novels; of neurotic plays dealing with people whose only weakness, *they* think, is that they are repressed; of literary studies whose whole thesis is that the American novel has always been afraid of sex? What is wrong with such works is not that the single points they make are incorrect, but that they rely upon a single point for a positive philosophy of life. It is impossible to write well and deeply in this spirit of Sisyphus, pushing a single stone up the mountain. It is impossible to write well if you start from an arbitrary point of view, and in the face of everything that is human, complex, and various, push home your *idée fixe*. It is impossible for the haunted, the isolated, the increasingly self-absorbed and self-referring self to transcend itself sufficiently to create works of literature.

Literature grows out of a sense of abundant relationships with the world, out of a sense that what is ugly to everyone else is really beautiful to you, that what is invisible to many men is pressingly alive and present to your writer's eye. We can no longer, by taking thought, transcend the life that consists in taking thought. The English novelist and philosopher Iris Murdoch has recently helped clear the air of desperate self-pity by saying that "We need to return from the self-centered concept to the other-centered concept of truth. We are not isolated free choosers, monarchs of all we survey, but benighted creatures sunk in a reality whose nature we are constantly and overwhelmingly tempted to deform by fantasy. Our current picture of freedom encourages a dream-like facility; whereas what we require is a renewed sense of the difficulty and complexity of the moral life and the opacity of persons."

By now the self-centered mind fashioned by Romanticism, constantly keeping itself open only to adjurations of absolute freedom and spontaneity, has traveled about as far along the road of self-concern as it can; it has nothing to discover further of itself but fresh despair. The immediate proof of this is in the quality of so much of the literature that has been shaped by Freudianism — only because all other creeds have failed it. It is not possible to write well with one's own wishes as the only material. It is not possible any longer to think anything out without a greater reality than oneself constantly pressing one's words into dramatic shape and unexpected meaning. All our words now are for our own emotions, none for the world that sustains the writer. And this situation is impossible, for it was never the self that literature was about, but what transcended the self, what comes home to us through experience.

Illness and Artistic Creativity

CLEMENS E. BENDA, M.D.

O VER the centuries, no doubt many great artists have
   fallen ill, but no record is at hand to indicate whether
their illnesses had a significant influence on their creativity. It was only in the nineteenth century that the illnesses of two contemporaries, Friedrich Nietzsche and
Vincent van Gogh, both of whom spent considerable time
in mental hospitals, gave rise to the question of how their
illnesses were related to their work.

"The more I become decomposed," wrote van Gogh in
one of his letters, "the more sick and fragile I am, the
more I become an artist." Few painters have been so artic-
ulate in their expression, and few men have so much insight into their own conditions.

Characteristic of his "mental attacks" was an intensification of his imagery. This intensification of perception occasionally came over van Gogh in the midst of
his work and brought about his representation of inner
visions, which assumed a new reality. He found it surprising that he, as modern man who admired Zola, the
Goncourts, and modern naturalism, was subject to spells
wherein religious ideas assumed a reality previously

recorded only by the great religious mystics. He observed the landscape with an emotional depth in which the objects of his perception and his own experience fused together into a new reality, but the experienced bliss was often interrupted by anxiety and fear.

The greatest intensity of van Gogh's work fell in the year 1888; forty-six of one hundred and eight major paintings were done in that year, whereas before 1887 there were only twelve. His work decreased after the acute onset of his illness, and somewhat fewer pictures are recorded for 1889 and 1890 than for 1888. Through his letters, we have an accurate account of the change in attitude which took place in the transition from impressionism to his new expressionistic style. In one letter he remarks, "Instead of reproducing exactly what I see, I use the colors arbitrarily in order to express myself more vigorously. I exaggerate the blonde of the hair. I arrive at orange colors, chrome, and light lemon yellow. Behind the head, in place of the ordinary wall of a common room, I paint the infinite. I achieve a background of purest blue, the strongest that I can express, and in this way the blonde radiant head achieves a mystical effect on the background of rich blue like a star in the deep azure. I am groping to find simpler and simpler techniques which may be not impressionistic. I would like to paint so that everyone who has eyes can see with complete clearness. Alas, I call this 'simplicity of technique.' "

With van Gogh's case, the problem of the artist and psychiatry suddenly moved into the public eye. Van Gogh's relationship between the artist and science and raises a testifies to the possibility of a warm and understanding relationship between the artist and science and raises a number of interesting questions. Is illness a factor in modern art? Does sickness support or suppress the creative process? Can van Gogh's painting be explained in any way by his illness? Do diagnosis and treatment of mental illness contribute to the understanding of the arts?

Since van Gogh's time, a number of great artists, among them the Norwegian painter Edvard Munch, have been known to suffer from mental disturbances. In our age of neurosis, when it is almost a prerequisite to be neurotic if one is to share in the cultural achievement of our times, the relationship between creative art and psychiatry has become even closer.

Munch's history in many points resembles that of van Gogh. Born in 1863 as the son of an army surgeon, he spent his childhood in Oslo. His mother died of tuberculosis when he was only five, and his oldest sister, who had been very close to him, also died of tuberculosis, when he was fourteen years old. Munch's haunting paintings of deathbeds and illness reproduced time and again the impact of these early experiences. Moreover, after the death of his mother, his father turned to religion in a way which was frightening to the children. As an old man, Munch recalled that his father "had a difficult temper, exhibited nervousness with periods of religious anxiety which could reach the borders of insanity as he paced back and forth in his room praying to God. . . . Disease and insanity were the black angels on guard at my cradle. . . . In my childhood I felt always that I was treated in an unjust way, without a mother, sick, and with threatened punishment in Hell hanging over my head."

Munch was frequently ill during childhood, and poor health often interrupted his attendance at school. At the age of twenty-seven, he was for the first time in a hospital, in France, for several months. From 1892 until 1908 he spent most of his time in voluntary exile abroad, mostly in Berlin, where he gained great success and recognition. In 1908 he had a "complete nervous collapse," culminating in excessive drinking, which led him into a sanitarium. The crisis which obsessed Munch found its most vivid expression in his painting called *Marat's Death*, in which the theme of Samson and Delilah is taken up and interpreted in the massive dead body of a man lying with the head toward the left lower edge, while the woman stands "erect and rigid, pressing her arms against her sides, excluding every feeling but that of her own self-justification expressed by the frozen and obsessive determination of her face."

Munch lived his last thirty years in solitude on the outskirts of Oslo, restricting his contacts to a few close friends.

The cases of van Gogh and Munch, as well as those of their respective literary contemporaries Nietzsche and Strindberg, prove beyond doubt that illness as such does not necessarily produce creativity, but often destroys the creative process. Moreover, the various forms of mental disturbance have very different effects upon different artists. Illness can give man a detachment and a courage which the average person does not command. Many artists have broken through the narrow bars of conventionality because of illness and have reached new frontiers which could never have been attained without it. An advancing illness often intensifies anxiety and dread, with a resultant increase in creative output. In van Gogh, the intensification of perceptual experience gave his vision a depth and color of unheard-of power. In Munch, on the other hand, illness caused suspicious withdrawal from friends, with a progressive narrowing of his experience.

When psychiatry became a biological science, scientists as well as the public confused the sick artist's work with his illness and denounced his paintings as fever-sick hallucinations, the output of a morbid mind. Many rather embarrassing studies of a pseudoscientific character are on record. But, in general, this period of psychiatric adventures has now come to an end. With the dawn of psychoanalytical investigations, a new approach to the artist was made. Interest was centered on the unconscious.

Since unconscious dynamics play a very important role in all creative achievements, it is not surprising that works of art attracted psychoanalytical attention. Freud himself did not expect too much from the study of mental illness, but thought that psychoanalysis would unearth significant themes in the work of great painters and writers. His controversial studies of Leonardo da Vinci, of Michelangelo's *Moses,* and of Dostoevsky have been equally acclaimed and rejected. Some of his minor disciples could not resist applying the analytical knife to the works and personalities of great artists, and many slipped into the pitfall of identifying creativity with neurosis, concluding that creativity stems from only partially successful sublimation of an unresolved Oedipus complex.

A number of psychoanalytical studies of artists are based on the theory that visual curiosity and the infantile urge to ask questions persist in the artist and philosophical thinker, that the artist continues in an infantile fixation, instead of living like ordinary human beings and taking for granted what life has to offer. One famous analyst wrote that creative people "stop at those early problems of life which give the child cause to ponder: the problems of birth and death, good and evil, aim and purpose of one's own existence." The creative artist and philosopher "ponders life instead of living it," thus failing to achieve a successful "sublimation of his infantile interests and inquisitiveness. [He] reveals by his endless doubting, searching, struggling that he is never done with the primary problems and suffers from them all his life."

Although the artist is credited with an ability to express his unconscious wealth of fantasy in a manner that "gives pleasure to himself and others," such achievement is said to be due to narcissism, interpreted as a kind of self-love concentrated on one's own personality, such as can best be observed in children. On this basis, the creative person lives only for self and concentrates on his ego and his work.

In evaluating the creative process as narcissism, inhibition, and failure to adjust to reality, psychoanalysts have made a serious mistake. Many an artist has feared that psychoanalysis might rob him of his creativity and produce a well-adjusted haberdashery salesman. The confusion between creativity and neurotic inhibition of creative expression unfortunately still exists in artistic circles and in psychiatric literature.

In an industrialized society, adjustment to reality is the main theme of mental health programs, and the best adjustment is often identified with sexual and financial successes. In the light of such ideas, many artists appear as victims of their own mother and father complexes. Not only does the world look down on artists as outsiders who are incapable of social adjustment, but the artists themselves are guilt-ridden and full of anxiety. It is regrettable that psychoanalysis has often reinforced their guilt feelings by overemphasizing the neurotic aspects of their conflicts. Jung and his school have generally avoided these pitfalls and have centered their attention on different aspects of the creative unconscious, achieving considerable understanding of mystic and primitive art.

To understand the relationship between illness and creativity, one must analyze the essence of creativity and study the effect of pathogenic influences on it. Fortunately, some scientific data are now available. Dr. Charles Hersch and Dr. Leslie Phillips, psychological researchers at Worcester State Hospital in Massachusetts, have used the conceptual framework of Professor Heinz Werner of Clark University and some of Dr. Anne Roe's earlier material on artists in an investigation comparing the creative mind with the average mind and with that of the schizophrenic patient. For the creative group they used a sample of eminent painters who have achieved national recognition.

In interpreting the Rorschach ink-blot test, the answers are scored in various categories according to whether movements, forms, colors, or other aspects determine the created image. This enables the psychologist to gain insight into the relative strength of various pressures within the individual and thus understand how he perceives the world and reacts to it. Certain types of answers are considered mature and indicate a high degree of integration, while others suggest emotionality and primitive diffuse emotionalism. Traditional interpretation of the Rorschach test did not permit discovery of creative aspects in the personality, and the misinterpretation of certain types of answers as primitive or regressive added to the confusion. The new study assumes that the creative personality does not operate at a fixed level of function but, rather, varies in its level of performance.

Creativity requires a constant reorganization which

cannot be achieved without constant fluctuation or mobility between progressive integration and regressive starting anew. Thus, creativity is a biphasic process. The creative artist has to command a flexibility which enables him to differentiate fixed configurations and reorganize the elements in nonexisting new patterns of imagery. And the creative person needs a greater ability to integrate those processes which we identify with maturity, as well as the more primitive personality patterns which enable him to regress and identify with objects on a rather primitive level. These primitive aspects of artistic personalities have often been confused in psychology with primitivity, infantilism, or schizophrenic lack of ego boundaries.

In an era when the unconscious and primitive patterns were the sole object of interest, artists were confused with neurotics and psychotics, who have only this aspect of creativity but lack the formative integration and real creative power. What especially distinguishes the great artist from the average person, and, even more, from neurotic inefficiency and schizophrenic decomposition? Artists give more mature, form-dominant responses than average people do, and both give significantly more integrative responses than the schizophrenics do. On the other hand, artists have more primitive responses than the average on what have been called "primitive" scores, but the artist's is a different type of primitive response from the schizophrenic's. Artists excel in the physiognomic responses of both groups.

The investigation showed that artists have a high percentage of mature responses of a specific nature, including movement conceptions, form-dominant responses, and primitive thought responses. The nature of their responses indicates that a creative personality is able to shift back and forth between self and environment. First, the boundaries between self and environment can be readily relaxed in a mode of identification. On the other hand, the boundaries are readily reinstated, with self and environment maintaining discrete and polar differentiation.

This research gives new insight into artistic creativity. Creative personalities have greater abilities than ordinary people for both progression and regression in their dealings with the world around them, but the regression in artistic creativity has no connection with the infantile regression of neurosis or mental illness.

Another fruitful source for a new interpretation of artistic creativity and for the understanding of the influence of illness on the artist has been the experimental production of temporary abnormal or psychotic conditions which subside after a few hours but give the physician an opportunity to observe the subject of the experiment and the subject an opportunity to record the alterations in his own experiences. In connection with Dr. Max Rinkel, I worked with one of the most outstanding Boston painters, who volunteered for two experiments, with lysergic acid and mescalin, respectively, because of his great interest in perceptual phenomena. Here are some excerpts from the observations of the two attending psychiatrists, as well as the self-experience of the painter.

8:20 A.M. Artist takes 60 mg. LSD. Thirty minutes later, feels a little drunk, slight tremor in the left hand. Five minutes later becomes happier, "the effects get stronger. I feel intoxicated." The tremors come and go in waves, spread over both hands. There is a euphoric mood, and A. gets more talkative, makes notes in his book, "intoxication, increased self-consciousness." Thirty minutes later, "changes in sensation of mouth and taste." At 9:28, "When I shift my eyes, everything seems brighter in color," has sensations in tongue, funny taste, more saliva. At 9:37, sensations of lighter color, values appear, the dark colors look the same. Feels extreme intoxication, momentarily pleasant sensations, but feeling more and more removed as waves come and go. At 9:48 feels "more detached" from himself. His writing changes, contractions of words occur, like "perctly" instead of "perfectly." Two minutes later the speech changes, too. He has different sensations of space, can see wider angles, everything looks smaller. At 10:18 starts a picture of Dr. R. "This has to be a caricature, not a likeness." "Hanging skin. You must have been very fat before." "Eyes: old woman's look; interesting eye structure." After two minutes of drawing very happily, "I am not sorry for you, I am sorry for me." The sensations of space come and go in waves, and space appears alternately removed and nearer. At 10:30 he talks slowly, feels in a "trancelike state," starts picture of Dr. R. At 10:46 he sits happily and draws, says little, has the sensation of "rapture," and says, "I could snap out but don't want to." At 10:53 feels great excitement. "I could go off in complete fantasy, can't move around, no feeling of awareness, sensation of floating." He scribbles, and his drawings become more and more disconnected. His pen gets arrested, and he makes dots instead of lines, looks at his pictures, smiles, "This is nothing." At 11:04 looks at his fountain pen, "This is like a telegraph pole"; looks at his hands and sees them detached in space. At 11:21, a new picture of Dr. R. Looks at him as "a new man, etheric colors, luminosity itself, feeling of spring, a much younger man." At 11:24 says to Dr. R., "You take on expressions I feel. You feel spasms?" Has strong sensations of empathy, is completely absorbed in Dr. R. "There is alarming identity between you and me." At 11:35 feels great buoyancy. "I am glad I am a painter." At 11:40 starts another drawing of Dr. R., draws from memory. "I hate to look away from paper. We have gotten off your portrait." Feels great "efficiency," is euphoric, "I care less." But the drawing itself does not progress, and he continues to draw one eye while the rest of the picture is not completed. At 11:52 feelings of ecstasy overcome him, he draws claws of birds, monsters; calls his drawing "monstrous, bizarre, exfoliations." At 12:17 experiences feelings of increased meaningfulness. Every gesture, every line acquires a great meaning. "I feel floating away." Looks into space and feels objects moving closer and farther away. Feelings of empathy and identity with his surroundings. The state of transformation persists for about an hour. The top of a head is missing, roaming about masked; laughing sensation. At 12:45, "Too bad to disrupt the sensations, pleasurable feelings, transformation of faces. I always try to hypnotize myself, have never succeeded." All colors in room have a light pastel coloring. . . . At 2:15 the perception of colors is much increased. Looks at the tablecloth, where there are some reflections from candelabra on ceiling. "Never noticed this before. Violet light with yellow aura around." At 2:30 the feelings of unreality come in waves, "state of turmoil, no order; chaotic is a better word than turmoil."

In his own studio, A. experiences the colors more intensely, "as if I noticed them for the first time." Tries to play his guitar, "It's tuned, I think." He has difficulties with coordination of his hands, but "I hear better. Sounds pleasant; Gee, I love the sounds," but the difficulties in playing increase. "I feel stiffer in playing." Calls the music "even nicer, sweeter, more human. Identification with sound of instrument is more complete." Complains that his mind wanders off, looks around with suspicion: "you people, destroying possibility of enjoyment." Around 3:00 is annoyed by our presence, "could otherwise enjoy myself," is suspicious, "You are not participating. I see it from your expressions." Feels suspicion arise, resentment. "You provoke something. Some people don't like this music. You provoke me to hostile reactions." After 3:15 the effect of the drugs is gradually petering out. "I am not feeling half as chaotic as in the restaurant." Feeling wears off. His hands appear to him clammy, moist, cyanotic. His suspiciousness is strong, and he draws monsters and animals. His attention comes and goes. At 4:00 the normal condition is restored, but waves of feelings of unreality are still coming and going at intervals.

These observations are very revealing. In one of his articles, research psychiatrist Max Rinkel summarized a number of his experiments at the Massachusetts Mental Health Center:

> The clinical manifestations depended essentially upon the amount of LSD administered. . . . Disturbances of thought processes and distortions of perception were quite common; other manifestations were related to behavior, affect, and mood. Hallucinations, illusions, and delusions did occur occasionally. Depersonalizations, suspiciousness, and paranoid reactions were frequently observed. The occurrence of hostility, often associated with extrapunitive or intrapunitive anger, was made the object of a special study and resulted in the observation (among others) that when the subject was hostile, he tended to devaluate the object, "a diabolical face," "a young woman looking one hundred years old"; but when the subject's attitude was affiliative, he tended to overvaluate the object, "big, my very rock of Gibraltar," or "glowing with youth and health."

Rorschach tests corroborated clinical observations and demonstrated the subjects' reduction in organization and integration, loss of emotional control, decrease in orientation to past and future. Anxiety and tension were increased in some individuals and decreased in others, with no consistency for either trend. The individuals apparently were aware of the fact that the LSD experiences were temporary, and insight remained preserved in spite of the drastic intellectual and emotional changes. I wish to stress one thought that bears out observations about the creative personality reported above: the intoxication of the schizogenic agent intensified the inner experiences but broke down the synthetic control functions and reduced the creative expression to doodling and fragmentation of lines. There is a conspicuous discrepancy between the experience of might and grandeur on the one hand and reduction of expressive facilities on the other.

The great artist represents the rare combination of strong unconscious drives with a strange power of controlled and mature integration of experience and the ability to express such order in symbolic forms of painted imagery or poetry. Studies of the unconscious alone will often find the painter near the neurotic, and even schizophrenic, with whom he may share tendencies to daydreaming and increased imagery formation; but in contrast to the ineffectiveness of the neurotic, the artist has strong forces of integration, control, and creativity at his disposal. It is this ability to transform the imagery into symbolic forms that distinguishes the artist from his less favored contemporaries.

Modern psychiatry recognizes the cognitive conscious and creative forces in man as that human attribute which enables him to transcend his emotional impressions and to be the creator of an inner world. Psychiatry can help reinforce and integrate the creative abilities and eliminate those fixations which inhibit the free shift between primitive and mature integrative functions. The painter needs identification in empathy and intuition, but at the same time needs the ability to withdraw and fall back on his own self-differentiation. In the neurotic we often find the anxious defense of one aspect of being. Some people never achieve a strong personality structure because the ego boundaries are too fluctuant. In others, the structure is rigid and compulsively petrified, and these people are never able to reorganize themselves and start anew with unprejudiced attitudes.

Man does not live in a reality common to all; each person lives in his own world, reflected in his imagery. To create this imagery in visual and literary forms, sharable by the creator and beholder alike, is the problem of all great art. In this way the artist and thinker moves again into the center of a civilization. If psychiatry succeeds in making the "outsider" again the true "insider," the representative of the best in humanity, it will serve the contemporary world in a manner previously denied to medicine.

The Nature of the Conflicts Between Psychiatry and Religion

ROYDEN C. ASTLEY, M.D.

————•◦•————

FOR several decades, but particularly since 1945, when the horrors and the problems of nuclear weapons exploded upon mankind, there has been in the United States a growing interest in religion and in psychiatry. Of particular concern to many has been the fostering of better relations between the two, often with a view to their joining forces, which it is hoped will lessen anxiety and suffering, and strengthen men and women in purposes deemed valuable to God and to humanity. This movement toward cooperation has supporters from psychiatry and from religion as well as from many other fields and walks of life. An example of its sincerity and serious endeavor may be seen in such an organization as the Academy of Religion and Mental Health, which was formed in 1956 and now has sixty chapters in fifty-seven cities, with a national membership of twenty-seven hundred, as well as one hundred and sixty affiliated institutions and organizations.

It seems to me that in their desire for closer cooperation and for collaboration — even for unity — some who

participate in the movement may remain unaware of sa-
lient differences between the psychiatric and the religious
views, or that in their enthusiasm they may lose sight of
those differences and of certain basic conflicts that continue to exist between the two. I believe that no good can
come of ignoring, glossing over, or minimizing those differences and conflicts. Rather, they should be clarified as
precisely and responsibly as possible, for nothing in the
human condition can be bettered by perpetuating ignorance or error. Not everyone will welcome such a clarifica-
tion, and some, to my regret, may be distressed; so that
what I shall be attempting is neither a simple nor an easy
task.

Let me begin by saying why statements of precision are
difficult to make, and at the same time give an example,
superficial but troublesome, of one aspect of the conflicts
between the two disciplines. The fact is, words themselves, even with the help of the best dictionaries, mean
or connote different things to different professional
groups. Anxiety, for example, to a psychoanalyst means
an unpleasant affect (feeling tone), accompanied by or
expressed via certain visceral, sensory, motor, and ideational phenomena, closely resembling fear, and due to a
damming up of energy in the psychic apparatus out of
unconscious concern lest its expression (in action, words,
or even thought) result in injury or loss of love. By no
means all psychiatrists would find this an acceptable definition, and a clergyman might well be intensely perplexed
by it. Indeed, a clergyman might possibly say that anxiety
is a state of apprehension, with bodily and mental expressions, signaling the agitation of a sinful soul by the Holy
Spirit — a definition with which not all clergymen would
agree, and which would certainly not suit the psycho-

analyst. To cite another example in the same vein, I once was present when a professor of physiology, a profoundly religious and prayerful man, heard a clergyman say he thought that extrasensory perception was bunk. The professor asked, "You don't believe in answered prayer?"

When it comes to such words as *love, conscience, soul,* and *truth,* troubles multiply. So much for the semantic sources of conflict and misunderstanding.

Since the psychoanalyst has already been mentioned, he ought forthwith to be properly placed in the psychiatric picture. In this country there are more than a thousand psychoanalysts who are formally recognized as being qualified, and of these all but a score or so are psychiatrists. Nowadays, the specialized training of the psychiatrist commences after he has earned his M.D., and after at least one year of internship in a general hospital. It consists of a minimum of three years of work as a resident physician, during which time he follows an approved program of study in psychiatry, and of bedside and office work, under supervision. (Often, following the residency, further time is devoted to additional training — for instance, in child psychiatry or in psychoanalysis.) After the residency, two more years of work in his specialty make him eligible to take examinations given by the American Board of Psychiatry and Neurology, and thus to earn his diploma in psychiatry. Such residency training is necessary also for membership in the American Psychoanalytic Association. In addition, membership in the latter requires a thoroughgoing personal analysis, upwards of one hundred and fifty hours of supervised work with patients, and four or more years of classes. All this work follows the residency and takes about seven years, during which time the student analyst earns his living in the practice of psychiatry. To sum up: the psychoanalyst is usually a psychiatrist who has gone on to become a specialist in psychoanalytic therapy.

Although the number of psychoanalysts in the United States today amounts to less than 7 per cent of the psychiatrists, psychoanalysis in less than seventy years has had a tremendous effect on American psychiatry; and despite developments in other areas — for example, drug therapy — it will in my opinion continue to exert its influence.

By this time the reader must have suspected correctly that I myself am an analyst. What, then, is the framework from which the analyst views the conflicts between psychiatry and religion? To define this framework, I must describe very briefly the origins and development of psychoanalysis.

During the nineteenth century, medicine, including psychiatry, adopted the scientific method as its ideal. This has resulted, during the last hundred years, in the accumulation of a vast amount of data relating to the anatomy, chemistry and physiology of the brain and the nervous system, and in the ability to detect, treat, and prevent certain disorders, such as the psychoses that may result from syphilis, from certain poisons, from vitamin and hormone deficiencies, and from tumors. In brief, many mental disorders resulting from organic changes are now controllable. Another group of illnesses, however, has not as yet yielded to the organic approach — for example, the hysterias, the obsessive-compulsive and manic-depressive disorders, the schizophrenias, and the character and personality disorders — although there are diligent psychiatric researchers who continue to seek an organic basis for them.

Prominent in the late nineteenth century were cases of hysteria, and those so afflicted moved from neurologist to neurologist, seeking relief.* As I have intimated, no rational diagnostic or therapeutic approach was available; but it was the destiny of one of the neurologists of the time, Sigmund Freud, who was stimulated by certain observations of Breuer, Bernheim, Charcot, and Liébault, his contemporaries in neurology, to concern himself not with the organic, but instead with the ideational and emotional material that the hysterical patient presented. Thus, for the first time, the scientific method was applied, by a physician thoroughly grounded in its use, to thoroughgoing research on the *psychological* processes of hysterical patients.

It is the history of mankind that not only does pain stimulate a search for surcease, but experiences encountered in the search are a chief source of knowledge. This is especially true in medicine, where the investigation of illness leads to an awareness of processes in the healthy which would never otherwise be suspected or investigated. We would never, for example, have achieved our understanding of the complex endocrine interactions involved in the menstrual cycle without the stimulus afforded by the distress of patients with gynecologic disorders.

* The neurologist is a doctor of medicine who has specialized in diseases of the tissues of the nervous system. In the past it was natural that both his colleagues and the public should turn to him for information and help in regard to mental disorder, as a stomach specialist might have been consulted regarding loss of appetite. Today, some neurologists are also trained in psychiatry, and a few in psychoanalysis.

This same serendipitous effect soon made its appearance as the data of the researcher-therapist Freud were collected. What he learned (I put it with almost ridiculous brevity) was that the symptoms of his hysterical patients could be understood in terms of their representing inadequate and abortive expressions of sexual strivings, of which the patients were quite unaware; that the patient, willy-nilly, tended presently to direct these strivings, however inappropriately, toward the analyst; that the patient was most painfully reluctant to permit himself to recognize and to acknowledge these strivings; that his reluctance and resistance stemmed from enormously distressing fears of injury or of being repudiated, fears which suggested he felt himself to be a bad child in the presence of a condemning adult; that indeed his sexual strivings *had* originated in and been a part of his childhood, and had involved him in loves, hates, fears, guilts and shames too oppressive to be borne, and thenceforth somehow put out of his mind by a thorough and enduring but mysterious process of deletion;* that in the throes of this painful childhood period of development not only was awareness of the sexual strivings censored, but attitudes were set, character traits laid down, and patterns of behavior formed. Freud learned further that if the sufferer sought psychoanalytic treatment, then, through the technique of free association, an interpersonal relation with the analyst developed that led to a revivifying of the hidden childhood problems. As the patient gradually discerned the significance of his symptoms, he was in a position to replace them by more appropriate and adult mechanisms of gratification or renunciation (of the hitherto unrecognized strivings), with accompanying changes to-

* In psychoanalytic terms, *repression*.

ward maturity in attitudes, character and behavior. As he was freed from his unconscious problem, the hysterical patient's symptoms would disappear and in due course he was cured.

I should add that as psychoanalytic experience and theory developed, it became apparent that primitive impulses other than the overtly sexual — for instance, anger, cupidity, and the wish to exploit — could also be expressed in symptoms. Psychoanalysis also began to understand and treat disturbances other than hysteria.

It took Freud years to accumulate his data and to work out his hypotheses and theories. His discoveries astounded him, although — and this was fortunate — they dismayed him less than they did his colleagues. These findings demanded a totally revised view of love and sexuality, of hatred and aggressiveness, of the nature of anxiety, of the sources of guilt and shame, of the ways in which attitudes develop and the emotional life grows, of how conscience and character are formed, and of how social behavior of the individual and the group is motivated. A very large order, indeed!

Prior to Freud, there was no body of data available to science, to medicine, or to psychiatry upon which to base a coherent (I do not say complete) theory of personality development or of behavior. Psychiatry *as a discipline* was therefore unable to take a point of view in this regard, and individual psychiatrists subscribed to whatever hypotheses or positions appealed to them. These might be materialistic or idealistic; humanistic or theologic; liberal, orthodox, or heterodox; eclectic, skeptical, or syncretic.

Now, it is very important to note that psychiatry, as a discipline, is still in precisely the same position today; *for it has not based itself on Freud's data and theories as, for example, biology has based itself on Darwin's contributions.** It subscribes to no coherent theory of personality development or behavior. It simply subscribes, along with the rest of medicine, to the scientific method as an ideal, and hence is in the same position vis-à-vis religion as is any other scientific discipline — astronomy, chemistry, or physics. Science deals only in observation and deduction; it can say nothing about what it cannot observe. Religion, on the other hand, deals with concepts of things that cannot be observed: God, the soul, Satan, angels, immortality, heaven, hell, resurrection. When I speak of religion I mean an institutionalized system of beliefs and practices, based upon faith, concerned with man in his relation to God, and claiming a position of central importance in the life of man and society. *Clearly, the basic orientations to man of psychiatry and of religion are poles apart, and their approaches to their problems are utterly dissimilar.*

It should also be clear that psychiatry, which cannot deal with what it cannot observe, has no competence to comment on many of the concepts of religion. But a further and less familiar point is implicit in this discussion: since psychiatry, as a discipline, has no coherent view of man, it has no rational basis for argument regarding the conclusions of religion as to the nature of personality and the sources of behavior. Psychiatry can account for neither; therefore some psychiatrists accept theological explanations while others reject them.

The position of psychoanalysis vis-à-vis religion is entirely different, for psychoanalysis does have — or at

---

* Psychiatry frequently borrows — piecemeal — from psychoanalysis.

least believes it has — a coherent view of man. During the past half-century, the data observed by Freud were repeatedly encountered in analytic therapy and in personal experience, and the basic aspects of his doctrine appeared to be validated. Furthermore, observations made upon the healthy, upon peoples of differing cultures, and upon the myths, literature and arts of mankind, have tended strongly to support many of Freud's findings. Here then *is* a coherent theory of personality development and behavior, able to account for much that was hitherto shrouded in mystery or explained in an entirely unscientific fashion. Let me recapitulate some of the implications of Freud's discoveries: they demanded a totally revised view of love and sexuality, of hatred and destructiveness, of the nature of anxiety, of the sources of guilt and shame, of the ways in which attitudes develop and the emotional life grows, of how conscience and character are formed, and of how social behavior of the individual and of the group is motivated.

There were further implications. The evidence grew that in psychology, as in embryology, the growing young recapitulate the development of the race. Indications gathered that social and cultural institutions, however useful or not useful, are expressions of the creativity of the unconscious — for example, that the monarchial form of government is a political expression of the child's view of the family with the powerful father at the head. There have been, of course, matriarchal cultures; and there is, as analysts (and many parents) know, a stage in the life of the child when he assumes that his mother is the all-powerful figure around which the entire family, including the father, revolves. Such simple, indeed oversimplified, examples serve to indicate the direction in which this new psychology was moving. Presently scientists of other disciplines, students of the arts and of literature, and theologians were all finding that psychoanalysis impinged upon their spheres. They had either to reject it or to revise their beliefs and practices.

Physiologists were faced with the fact that not only does physiology make psychology, but that psychology can alter physiology — and psychosomatic medicine appeared. Sociology and anthropology were stimulated to far-reaching researches in terms not previously possible. The Greek and Elizabethan dramas — for example the *Oedipus Rex* of Sophocles, and *Hamlet* — were interpreted in a fashion that compellingly explained their universality and their deathless fascination. And religion, as an institutionalized system of beliefs and practices, came under analytic scrutiny, as persons in analysis furnished mounting evidence relating the origins of their religious impulses to the childhood need to maintain comfortable relations with their parents, whom they saw as all-powerful. Thus it appeared that psychoanalysis was threatening the very basis of religion by suggesting that the *image* of God was no more than a projection of certain aspects of the father, or the parents, as the child saw them. *Actually, psychoanalysis said nothing about the existence or the nature of God.* It only purported to throw new light on man and his beliefs, and his troubles and conflicts with them. However, the fact that Freud, who was personally an atheist, was the proponent of the analytic approach, strengthened the impression that psychoanalysis would seek to destroy religion. It has no such intention, but it does intend to understand man's psychology, and if hitherto cherished beliefs and practices of *any* sort — racial, social, familial, economic, political, personal, religious — are lost or changed in the process, that is the way it must be. Science has nothing against fantasy as such, but it is dead set against the confusion of fantasy with fact, and psychoanalysis holds to this position.

Let me pause again to recapitulate. Thus far we have encountered three sorts of conflict between psychiatry and religion. First, the semantic; second, the opposition between the scientific and deductive approach to problems of living and of existence and the revealed and inductive approach; and third, the direct threat to cherished religious beliefs and practices that comes from psychoanalysis.

Let us turn, now, to the relations between religion and psychiatry in the moral sphere. Religion, at least as it is conceived in Western culture, is a vehicle of moral and ethical values. These are usually considered to stem from the Deity, and the representatives of organized religion are regarded as arbiters and custodians of morals and ethics. Since psychiatry, as a discipline, has no coherent view of personality development or behavior, it has no pertinent statements to make about morality and ethics except to be in favor of "the good." But, again, psychoanalysis is in a different position. Just as the historian knows that most of the Decalogue preceded Moses (see the code of Hammurabi, *circa* 2000 B.C.), so the analyst has come to know that the origins of conscience and character belong far back in the first six years of childhood, and have to do with strictly human childhood problems of love and hate in the family. The beginnings are only that — beginnings. Later, accretions and elaborations and precipitations occur, but morality begins in childhood, and as a result of the child's psychological mechanisms. For example, the healthy small boy, in his strivings to take first place with his mother, resents his father and wishes him gone; but he also loves, admires, and needs his father. To resolve his problem, he takes over the parents' point of view (with father as proponent) that mother is father's woman, thus erecting a barrier within himself against impulses toward what adults call murder and incest. He does this not because he believes that murder, sex, and incest are morally wrong, but because he is weak, fearful, angry, needy, and loving. The moral position *follows* his renunciation; and it arises as a result of his pragmatism. No code, religion, deity, or clergyman is involved.

For some years after this *tour de force* the child will be, as it were, hypermoral, and will have, indeed, the appearance of sexual "innocence." This is because he will have put out of his mind something too oppressive to be borne. He will for a time treat sexual impulses as if they were dangerous — or, in moral terms, as wrong; and his pubescent urges, when they appear, will be experienced, to some extent at least, with anxiety, as if they and he were bad.

Observe, now, that to the pubescent child, virtue appears to lie in abstinence and vice in gratification — and this because he has still got the impulse and the object confused; for they were, years back, united in his early rivalrous yearnings for his mother, and they remain — the impulse and the object — connected in his unconscious. How shall this situation be viewed? Shall the child be supported in his view that abstinence is right, or shall he be supported in growth toward an appropriate outlet — at this age, masturbation? (You will note that it is his *growth* that is supported. He is *not* encouraged to mas-

turbate.) Here, clearly, there may arise a conflict between religion and psychoanalytic psychiatry involving a
"moral" question; for some religions and some proponents
of religion would be opposed to an acceptance of masturbation, deeming it wrong or sinful, while the analyst
would view it as a normal activity which may have, for
some time or for some people, inappropriate emotional
reverberations.

In the area of moral questions, there is a sharp difference between psychoanalysis and religion on three
scores, two of which have just been mentioned: the origins of morality and the content of the moral code (some
of the specific issues on which psychoanalysis and religion take different attitudes are sexual relations outside
marriage, divorce, contraception, relations with authority figures, freedom of thought). The *third* point of difference has to do with flexibility. Religion tends — please
note that I say *tends* — to deal in absolutes. It has shibboleths: saved and lost, chosen and not chosen. And this
tendency towards absolutism or authoritarianism is reflected in its somewhat inflexible formulation of codes
and in its often uncompromising adherence to them. The
analyst, seeing a different and human source of codes, is
a relativist, who seeks always to test the appropriateness
of the code to the reality situation. I shall give two examples.

A young man came to treatment suffering from
chronic anxiety, sleeplessness, and digestive upsets with
no discernible organic background. He was a gambler
and a cheat, as his father had been before him. Indeed,
the father had been a Fagin to his small son. One day my
patient came into the office almost in a panic. It presently

developed — and in the form of a confession — that his awful anxiety had to do with his having paid his check in a restaurant. Now let us not laugh, but rather understand: this man had actually been taught ways of avoiding payment and had been made to believe that only "dopes" paid up. On this particular day he had, in effect, rebelled shamefully against his conscience — that powerful father image from his childhood whose code he had adopted. My patient revealed himself to be the most "moral" of men: his panic was due to the fact that his code, which (as it should be) was so difficult to live up to in our society, was enforced from within by a cruelly harsh conscience. Make no mistake — he was not amoral; nor, in terms of his upbringing, immoral. On the contrary, he was inflexibly bound to an inflexible code that simply differed vastly in *content* from that of society or of any religious group. The analyst sees less dramatic cases frequently: for example, a man who could not read because reading was unconsciously equated with gratifying a childhood curiosity that his conscience forbade.

My second case has to do with a young man with an extremely rigid code of Christian ethics. He was referred for treatment when excruciating headaches were unexplained and unrelieved by diligent physicians using a somatic approach. It soon developed that in his work, his marriage, and his habits of life, he was being unwittingly submissive to cruel and rejecting (unconscious) parent images, out of fear of being entirely bereft of love. As his own sense that he could be loved increased, he left an overdemanding job and an overbearing superior, got a divorce from a carping and ungiving wife, and began to enjoy an occasional evening of beer with the boys. His headaches had become very infrequent and much less severe; and in due course he remarried, and lived comfortably — though with a few of the earmarks of the overworked "morality" that he had previously exhibited.

We have now discussed four areas of possible conflict between psychiatry and religion. But the list is not yet complete.

In speaking of cure, Freud explained that the goal of his treatment was to relieve the patient of his neurotic misery and to leave him with the ordinary unhappiness that is common to mankind. Three comments must be made about that statement. To begin with, problems of character and of somatic illness have frequently been shown to have a neurotic basis, and by now it is recognized as only half a joke when someone says, "Everybody's crazy, but the analysts are the only ones who know they are." Thus, Freud's remark applies to *many* more sick people than those with clear-cut neurosis. Secondly, the statement disavows happiness as a psychoanalytic value: no one should go to an analyst to achieve happiness! Third, it is implied that men can find ways to manage their essential unhappiness. There appear to be five resorts when all else has failed, as at times it must: drugs to dull the pain, work, enjoyment of art, religion, and interest in observing and experiencing one's own functioning. Drugs are, of course, a dangerous and potentially fatal surcease. Enjoyment of art is far less of a threat, but seems available to few, and may sink to a kind of masturbatory level. Work cannot be too long sustained in the face of fatigue and discouragement. Religion, based as it is upon faith, frequently seems to require too great a credulity and too much self-abnegation. Interest in observing and experiencing one's own functioning may isolate a man, or lead him to seek self-destructive experiences. And yet psychoanalysis implies that, though life is hard indeed, the game is worth the candle; and that with the aid of anodynes, taken in moderation and according to one's taste, one can live it with some satisfaction. A man can be free to know who he is, and what he is, and be responsible for himself and to himself.

Religion, mark you, takes an immensely different point of view. It is concerned in its essence with the relation of man to God, and claims a central position in life for this concern. (I do not suggest that it is not concerned with the relation of man to man, but that is not primary.) Only in relation to God, it says, can man know who he is and what he is; and he must be responsible to God. Since God is outside the realm of science, and since the image of Him has seemed to the analyst to have grown out of childhood needs and fantasies, the analyst, as such, has no way to agree or to disagree. He can only say, "Some see it that way." (He may, of course, as a private person, be religious.) At this point the levels of discourse are really different.

Now, a final point. Both psychiatry and religion are concerned with the relief of suffering. This would appear to create a bond. However, it seems to me a bond somewhat similar to that between a veterinarian and a lioness with a sick cub. The veterinarian is interested in the cub's healthy development into what he is destined to be: a vigorous, autonomous animal, no longer dependent on lioness or veterinarian. The lioness, for all her anxiety, wants her cub to be *her* cub. She has no vision of his autonomous future, and is fiercely possessive.

Some years ago the Marriage Council of Philadelphia wished to incorporate and to apply for a charter from the

Commonwealth, and its board sought the support of the County Medical Society and the Philadelphia Bar Association. There was a joint meeting, and after discussion the committee for the Bar Association rendered an opinion: Marriage is a legal contract, counsel is advice; the Marriage Council has no competence to give legal advice, is practicing law illegally, and should not be supported.

By the same token, the clergyman might take the view that marriage is a spiritual relationship, counsel is consultation with a view to advice, and the spiritual adviser is therefore the only proper marriage counselor. The psychiatrist, the psychoanalyst, the anthropologist, and the sociologist could all make similar possessive, proprietary, and competitive claims to be the appropriate authorities. The point I wish to make is that psychiatry and religion see problems differently, and see differing approaches and differing kinds of resolutions as optimal. There *is* competition and it should be recognized for what it is.

Analytic experience suggests that if a patient's religious beliefs and practices are intimately connected with his unconscious conflicts, they will be changed by *thorough* treatment. They may be strengthened, but that is not likely. *Where thoroughgoing treatment of neurosis is concerned,* religion is likely to lose many more adherents than it will gain, even though no competent analyst would think of attacking a patient's religion. The fact is that the patient, as he traces back (to their origins in childhood) the sources of his neurotic conflicts, is apt eventually to see his religious impulses in an entirely new light. However, a full analysis can be undertaken by only a small fraction of the population. Psychotherapy, while less thorough, is frequently of inestimable value to the patient and is unlikely to have any effect upon his religion.

To sum up: The nature of the conflicts between psychiatry and religion has been glimpsed in a number of areas, of which I have explored six.

First, semantic problems of serious dimensions present themselves at the outset. Much careful definition is required to dispel the mist that they engender.

Second, the approach of a science is skeptical, it deals only with what can be observed, and it knows no absolutes. The approach of religion is by faith, it deals with what cannot be observed, and it accepts — even insists upon — absolutes. Psychiatry, deriving from scientific medicine, thus differs from religion; but since psychiatry, as a discipline, has no scientific psychology, it is psychoanalysis which is most in conflict with the religious view of God and man.

Third, psychoanalysis asserts that man is mainly motivated or inhibited by his unconscious, and that the image of God and the relation to that image are traceable to childhood needs and fantasies that reside in the unconscious. Psychoanalysis says nothing about God's existence or His nature — these are beyond its competence, as they are beyond that of psychiatry.

Fourth, while psychiatry, as a discipline, has little or nothing to say about morality except to favor "the good," psychoanalysis sees morality as a pragmatic outgrowth of the child's emotional development, and is relativist as to the content and applicability of codes. Religion, on the other hand, sees morality as deriving from the commandments of the Deity, for man's benefit; finds its source and content in revelation; and tends to be not relativist but authoritarian and absolute.

Fifth, psychoanalysis sees man as capable not of sustained happiness, but of at least independently facing his own problems and achieving a sense of personal freedom and satisfaction in being autonomous. Religion sees man as a creature who, for a true sense of well-being, must come to depend unconditionally upon his Creator.

Sixth, a bond appears to exist in the mutual interest of psychiatry and religion in the relief of suffering. Psychiatry, as a discipline, still seeks a scientific understanding of many mental disorders and an organic method of treatment. Psychoanalysis, however, sees relief and health as stemming from awareness of and mastery over buried childhood fantasies and feelings, and in concomitant emotional growth. And religion offers surcease and health in terms of faith in and dependence upon God, and upon those expressions and experiences of God's interest and love that come to persons who seek after and trust Him, and who attempt to live as He would have them live.

I have not minced words, nor, I hope, blurred concepts; and I know I have not said easy things. It is my conviction that both psychiatry and religion are better served by honest confrontation of the conflicts between them than by fuzzy attempts to minimize their differences and to represent them as fellow travelers.

Readings in Psychiatry—A Selection for the Layman

A General Introduction to Psychoanalysis. SIGMUND FREUD. Paperback. Washington Square: 1960. Freud was a master of simple, lucid expression, and these elementary lectures are the classic primer on psychoanalysis.

An Outline of Psychoanalysis. SIGMUND FREUD. Norton: 1949. Freud's final, concise summation of his doctrines.

What Life Should Mean to You. ALFRED ADLER. Putnam's Capricorn Books: 1958. A comprehensive statement of Adler's views, liberally illustrated with case histories.

An Introduction to Jung's Psychology. FRIEDA FORDHAM. Paperback. Pelican: 1953. An able exposition of the theories of Jung, whose own writings are for the most part difficult and sometimes formidable.

The Basic Writings of C. G. Jung. Edited by VIOLET S. DE LASZLO. Modern Library: 1959. This representative selection from Jung's major works presents the structure of his thought, his views on therapy, and papers on psychology and religion.

Neurosis and Human Growth. KAREN HORNEY. Norton: 1950. Here Karen Horney, who founded her own school of psychoanalysis in the 1940s, makes a revealing analysis of the various mechanisms and patterns of neurotic behavior. Easy to understand and illuminating.

Oedipus: Myth and Complex. PATRICK MULLAHY. Hermitage Press: 1948. This overall survey of psychoanalytic theory and of the differences between the various schools is an able job of popularization. It presents clearly and succinctly the doctrines of Freud, Jung, Adler, Sullivan, Horney, Fromm, and Rank.

The Mind of Man. WALTER BROMBERG. Harper Torchbooks: 1959. A well-written history of psychotherapy. It covers mental healing throughout the ages, the mental health movement, psychoanalysis and its derivatives.

The Life and Work of Sigmund Freud. ERNEST JONES. 3 vols. Basic Books: 1953-1957. The definitive biography of the master by the most loyal of his disciples.

Psychiatry Today. DAVID STAFFORD-CLARK. Paperback. Pelican: 1952. An excellent all-around book on modern psychiatry. Lucid and well-written.

Mind and Body. FLANDERS DUNBAR. Random House: 1955. This straightforward, readable treatise on psychosomatic medicine has achieved widespread popularity. Recommended by the *Journal of the American Medical Association.*

Freud and The Twentieth Century. Edited by BENJAMIN NELSON. Paperback and hard cover. Meridian Books: 1957. A first-rate symposium containing sixteen essays on various aspects of the Freudian revolution. The range is broad, and the contributors are varied and distinguished.

Freud: The Mind of the Moralist. PHILIP RIEFF. Viking: 1959. A searching commentary on the entire range of Freud's thought. This is a book for readers already acquainted with psychoanalytic theory.

Practical and Theoretical Aspects of Psychoanalysis. LAWRENCE S. KUBIE. Praeger: 1960. A guide to present-day analytic procedures. Discusses candidly a number of the problems which arouse concern and criticism.

Freudianism and the Literary Mind. FREDERICK J. HOFFMAN. Louisiana State University Press: 1945. A well-written study of the influence of psychoanalysis on literature.

Art and Psychoanalysis. Edited by WILLIAM PHILLIPS. Criterion Books: 1957. Twenty-six essays on the application of psychoanalytic theory to the arts and the creative process. Among the contributors are Freud, Thomas Mann, Ernest Jones, Lionel Trilling, Edmund Wilson.

Life Against Death. NORMAN O. BROWN. Paperback. Modern Library: 1960. The author examines man's relation to culture and the psychoanalytic meaning of history. This book, already famous among students of psychoanalysis, is a brilliant but complex and difficult work — original, extreme, highly controversial.

The Hidden Remnant. GERALD SYKES. Harper: 1962. A well-written, unconventional commentary on the various schools of psychoanalysis and psychotherapy, which seeks to distill from them their most valuable insights.

Man's Search for Himself. ROLLO MAY. Norton: 1953. A thoughtful, readable book which examines the characteristic fears and conflicts of modern man. The author, a well-known New York psychotherapist, suggests ways of working toward a real awareness of self and of achieving integration.

Psychoanalysis and Religion. ERICH FROMM. Yale University Press: 1950. Dr. Fromm holds that neurosis is essentially the result of man's failure to develop his moral and spiritual potentialities. He distinguishes between the "authoritarian" and "humanistic" aspects of religion, attacking the former and defending the latter.

Notes on the Contributors

———————

DR. ROYDEN C. ASTLEY is director of the Pittsburgh Psychoanalytic Institute and professor of psychiatry at the University of Pittsburgh.

DR. CLEMENS E. BENDA, a Boston psychiatrist, is the author of several books and many articles on human development and creativity. His most recent work, *The Image of Love: Modern Trends in Psychiatric Thinking,* was published by the Free Press of Glencoe, Illinois.

BROCK BROWER, editor and writer, went to Oxford as a Rhodes Scholar and received his master's degree there in 1956. He has contributed articles on various aspects of the American scene to leading magazines in this country.

DR. STANLEY COBB, one of the most honored figures in American medicine, has been professor of neuropathology at Harvard, chief psychiatrist at the Massachusetts General Hospital, and president of the American Psychosomatic Society. His contributions run to five books and nearly three hundred monographs.

DR. ROBERT COLES, after graduating from Harvard and from Columbia's College of Physicians and Surgeons, took his psychiatric residence at the Massachusetts General Hospital and McLean Hospital. He then completed a period of special training in child psychiatry at Boston's Children's Hospital, and recently he served in the Air Force as chief of a neuropsychiatric center in Mississippi.

ALFRED KAZIN, well-known author and literary critic, has published essays on psychoanalysis which brought him an invitation to lecture to an audience of analysts. His most recent book, *Contemporaries,* was published last year by Atlantic – Little, Brown.

MIGNON McLAUGHLIN has been a frequent contributor to the *Atlantic Monthly* and other magazines. Her aphorisms, published periodically under the title "The Neurotic's Notebook," will eventually appear in book form.

O. HOBART MOWRER is professor of psychology at the University of Illinois. He has taught at Princeton, Yale, and Harvard, and in 1954 was president of the American Psychological Association. In recent years, he has published two technical volumes on the psychology of learning, and a paperback entitled *The Crisis in Psychiatry and Religion.*

DR. PETER B. NEUBAUER, an Austrian-born, Swiss-trained psychoanalyst, has worked since 1941 in New York. He has made the field of child psychiatry his specialty, and is director of the Child Development Center in Manhattan.

DR. MORTIMER OSTOW, a practicing psychoanalyst associated with New York's Montefiore Hospital, is the author of *Drugs in Psychoanalysis and Psychotherapy,* published by Basic Books.

PHILIP RIEFF, a sociologist, has taught at the University of Chicago and the University of California, and is at present on the faculty of the University of Pennsylvania. His latest book, *Freud: The Mind of the Moralist,* was published by Viking Press in 1959.

CHARLES ROLO, author, editor, and critic, was for many years associated with the *Atlantic Monthly.* A long-standing interest in psychoanalysis led him to embark on research for a book on the cultural impact of Freud, and he is serving on the board of trustees and executive committee of a psychoanalytic clinic in New York.

JOHN R. SEELEY was educated in Chicago and now teaches sociology and psychiatry at the University of Toronto.

He is co-author of *Crestwood Heights*, the first intensive psychological study of a North American community.

GERALD SYKES is a novelist, essayist, and student of the new psychology. His most recent book, *The Hidden Remnant*, published by Harper & Row in 1962, is a critical survey and sifting of the various schools of psychoanalysis and psychotherapy.

GREER WILLIAMS, assistant director of the Children's Hospital Medical Center in Boston, served for five years as director of information of the Joint Commission on Mental Illness and Health. He was editor of *Action for Mental Health*, the commission's report to Congress, published by Basic Books in 1961.

RUDOLPH WITTENBERG, a psychoanalyst engaged in private practice, is a consultant in psychotherapy to the City Hospital at Elmhurst and to the Mental Health Consultation Center in New York City. He is also on the faculty of the New School for Social Research. The most recent of his five books is *Common Sense about Psychoanalysis*, published by Doubleday in 1962 and now available in paperback.